Fiber Boost

Fiber Boost:

Everyday Cooking for a Long, Healthy Life

Amy Snider

KEY PORTER BOOKS

Dedicated to Mike,
Shelby and my sweetie, Gracie,
for the one that isn't finished yet.

Library and Archives Canada Cataloguing in Publication

Snider, Amy
    Fiber boost : everyday cooking for a long, healthy life / Amy Snider.

Includes index.
ISBN 1-55263-592-9

    1. High-fiber diet—Recipes. I. Title.

RM237.6.S54 2004   641.5'63   C2004-904158-4

The publisher gratefully acknowledges the support of the Canada Council for the Arts and the Ontario Arts Council for its publishing program. We acknowledge the support of the Government of Ontario through the Ontario Media Development Corporation's Ontario Book Initiative.

We acknowledge the financial support of the Government of Canada through the Book Publishing Industry Development Program (BPIDP) for our publishing activities.

Key Porter Books Limited
70 The Esplanade
Toronto, Ontario
Canada M5E 1R2

www.keyporter.com

Text design: Jack Steiner
Electronic formatting: Jean Lightfoot Peters

Printed and bound in Canada

04 05 06 07 08 5 4 3 2 1

Contents

Foreword

Fiber, You Say?

It wasn't so long ago that fiber was discussed in hushed tones and only when absolutely necessary. It fell into a category that prudish schoolmarms and prissy great-aunts warned kids was immodest for nice people to discuss openly. Those were also the days when white bread, canned peas and carrots and chicken à la king made frequent appearances on most middle-class dinner tables.

Today, fiber is acknowledged as an important element in our diets. Scientific research shows that fiber can help us maintain good health and prevent illnesses such as cancer and heart disease; research also indicates that eating an adequate amount of fiber can lead to a longer life. Yet studies show that few North Americans are eating as much of this nutrient as they should, despite improved access to fiber-rich ingredients at the grocer's.

Why is that? Probably because old habits die hard. Probably because many of us have not modified our cooking habits to ensure adequate fiber in our diets. Probably because busy people too often depend on fast-food outlets, where fiber-rich foods are rarely available or, if they are offered, are prepared in lackluster, unappealing ways. Probably because Amy Snider hadn't written this book yet.

I had the pleasure of taste-testing many of the recipes in *Fiber Boost* and was surprised by how good these fiber-rich recipes are. I expected to have to settle for foods that were good for me but tasted kind of blah. Instead, I was delighted to find that these recipes produced delicious meals—and I've found myself wanting to make them again and again. *Fiber Boost* features approachable, easy-to-follow recipes for foods we all like to eat, such as pasta, decadent desserts and even meat dishes. Amy Snider makes these favorites in new, healthier ways, and I predict that more people of all ages will soon be eating diets enriched with adequate amounts of fiber. It won't be because their doctors or the media tell them they should. It will be because Amy Snider's fiber-rich recipes will become family favorites they just have to make often.

—Dana McCauley

Introduction

Why a Book About Fiber?

When my publisher, Anna Porter, and I first sat down to discuss creating *Fiber Boost*, we agreed that this book should be filled with useful information about how fiber can contribute to good health and a long life. We also agreed that I should try to keep the topic light and, more specifically, to take the focus away from (pardon the expression) the "ins and outs" of the digestive system. My job is to make increasing fiber in our diet fun.

Fiber is a nutrient that needs attention. While evidence of its healthy benefits has become common knowledge, North Americans are consuming only about half the fiber recommended by health professionals. Most people grimace and groan when told to increase the fiber content of their diet. Terms like "roughage" and "regularity" do nothing to improve fiber's appeal to the younger generation. Yet despite its less than sexy image, fiber has a lot to offer people of all ages. Although I am still in my twenties, my nutrition background has taught me that the best way to age gracefully is to have a healthy lifestyle that includes regular physical activity and wholesome, nutritious foods. We all want to be active and vital throughout our lives, and a high-fiber diet can help us achieve this goal. Diets with adequate fiber have been linked to the prevention of several major diseases, such as heart disease and certain cancers. Also, fiber can be a valuable component of any weight-loss program.

In the past, fiber has been associated with managing the negative aspects of growing older. In fact, the very word evokes images of beans, bran and "Pass me the prune juice, Marge." Yet fiber should be considered one of the basics of healthy eating. It is found in many wonderful foods such as vegetables, fruits and whole grains.

That is why, in *Fiber Boost*, I have included fantastic, fuss-free recipes suitable for cooking every day to serve to your family or guests. This is a book for children as well as men and women, because it is never too early to learn to enjoy delicious wholesome foods that contain not only fiber but a wealth of other nutrients.

In the last half of the twentieth century, processed and packaged foods became ubiquitous. Immersed in an increasingly competitive workforce, people are scrambling when it comes to mealtimes. Convenience foods have inundated grocery-store shelves with instant "gourmet" dinners ready at the push of a microwave button. North Americans have become used to eating these "plastic foods," which are typically high in fat and full of simple carbohydrates. They are a quick fix, but in terms of nutritional content, convenience foods generally leave much to be desired, especially in their fiber content. Whole foods such as fresh vegetables and fruits, whole grains and legumes have been replaced in our diets with refined flour, shortening and preservatives.

Statistics show that over half the U.S. population is overweight, and Canadians aren't far behind. A national health survey done in the late 1990s reveals that 46 percent of Canadians are overweight or obese and are at increased health risk because of their weight. North Americans seem plagued with illnesses that stem from obesity. Meanwhile, in other parts of the world, populations whose diets are based on fiber-rich whole grains and vegetables are leading healthier lives.

Nevertheless, wellness is the trend of the new millennium, and many people are in search of total health makeovers. Detoxifying treatments are becoming increasingly popular, but a steady high-fiber diet eliminates the need for such drastic intervention. By gradually increasing the fiber content of your diet to the recommended levels, you will be well on the way to a healthy digestive tract. The positive benefits of this commitment will be felt in all aspects of your life: you will have more energy, sleep better and enjoy a general sense of well-being.

Studies have shown that eating 25 to 40 grams of fiber a day will have a positive impact on disease prevention and everyday vitality. But how can you be sure you are eating enough fiber? The recommended solution is often to adopt a vegetarian diet—a healthy idea but not an enjoyable one for many people. I don't believe it is necessary to go on a radical diet in order to eat more fiber. *Fiber Boost* contains recipes for meat-eaters who want to consume more fiber but don't want to give up their favorite meaty dishes. You can achieve a healthy balance without overhauling your entire lifestyle. Many of your favorite foods can have a fiber makeover, and the transition can be agreeable for everyone in your family. Instead of scrapping those classic family dishes, you can learn how to modify them into fiber-friendly recipes.

How to Use This Cookbook

The recipes in *Fiber Boost* are designed to be both healthful and a rich source of fiber. Each recipe contains a nutrient summary with information on how much fiber is in the recipe:

> *A source of fiber:* Contains at least 2 grams per serving.
> *A high source of fiber:* Contains at least 4 grams per serving.
> *A very high source of fiber:* Contains at least 6 grams per serving.

The nutrient summary also indicates when a recipe is an excellent source of other common nutrients, such as vitamin A, vitamin C, calcium and iron, and also gives information on sodium content. Those concerned about salt intake can eliminate the added salt from the recipes and substitute low-sodium broth for regular broth. Although the recipes are not specifically low-fat, I have generally incorporated heart-healthy fats such as olive and canola oil. For those who are concerned about fat intake, here are a couple of tips to cut out excess fat:

☐ Substitute skim-milk cheeses and low-fat dairy products in salads, side dishes and main-course recipes. (For baked goods, make substitutions only when indicated, because the fat content of the ingredient may be essential to the structure of the finished product.)
☐ Use nonstick skillets coated with nonstick spray to cut down on excess oil when sautéeing vegetables and meats.

Fiber Boost focuses on recipes featuring whole foods that can be found in your local supermarket. The recipes are delicious and appetizing but also straightforward and approachable. If you cannot find a particular ingredient, you may need to talk to the store's product manager or take a trip to a bulk-food store. I hope that you will enjoy the recipes in *Fiber Boost* and that you will take the ideas you learn here and apply them to all your favorite recipes for a healthy makeover. The Fiber Boosters charts on pages 9–11 and the Three-Week Fiber-Boosting Plan on page 132 will help you make the transition to fiber-rich cooking.

Defining Fiber

In the most basic of definitions, fiber is indigestible carbohydrate. Carbohydrates come from plant foods. Humans don't possess the enzymes needed to digest every part of the plants we eat. The chewing process breaks down food; after we swallow, it is broken down even further by the acids in the stomach, after which enzymes aid in the absorption of valuable nutrients. The body then eliminates what it can't use. As it is the structural base of all plants, fiber could be considered the box in which plant nutrients are delivered to the body. Historically, scientists dismissed the box, focusing only on the nutrients inside, but we are now beginning to realize that the container itself has an impact on our health. Experts are still learning about all the components of fiber that are beneficial to the body. Until more is known, it is best to simplify fiber into two major categories: soluble and insoluble.

Most people correctly link wheat bran, vegetable skins, seeds and nuts with fiber and stop there. These foods are sources of insoluble fiber. Insoluble fiber gets its fame from its ability to absorb water. It has a bulking effect and speeds the transit of food through your system. With consistent adequate intake of insoluble fiber, food waste is eliminated from the digestive system quickly and efficiently.

Soluble fiber is the other partner in a healthy digestive system. It is found in fruit pectin, some legumes, oats, barley and rye. As the name suggests, it dissolves in water, forming a gel that slows the movement of food, giving your body time to absorb key nutrients while carrying away less beneficial ones such as cholesterol. These two components of fiber work as a team to help you get the most out of your food and then move it out.

It is important to include both types of fiber in your diet. Rather than simply adding a supplement to your breakfast, choosing whole foods throughout the day is the best way to achieve a healthy balance. *Fiber Boost* offers delicious recipes and tips to help you accomplish a positive lifestyle change. But is important to make any dietary changes gradually. Because of the way fiber functions in your body, fiber-rich foods can cause some uncomfortable side effects, which may deter you from eating enough. To help you avoid discomfort, see the Three-Week Fiber-Boosting Plan on page 134 for advice on how to gradually increase fiber intake.

Drinking adequate water (even extra) as you eat more fiber is essential. Actually, instead of thinking of fiber as a partnership between soluble and insoluble, it really is more accurate to see it as a three-way interaction. Both types of fiber use the water available in your body, making it unavailable for other functions. Without adequate hydration, the soluble and insoluble fibers cannot perform their helpful tasks. This can lead to the uncomfortable side effects that we want to avoid. So remember to drink at least six to eight glasses of water per day. Watch your intake of caffeinated beverages such as coffee, tea and cola because they tend to cause dehydration. Limit your intake to no more than four cups per day.

And, as a precaution, consult your doctor before making any significant changes to your eating habits.

Fiber for Health and Disease Prevention

Fiber and Obesity

Statistics show that approximately 300,000 Americans die each year of weight-related illnesses, including heart disease, cancer and Type II diabetes. An alarming increase in childhood obesity is a disturbing predictor of future obesity. Children who suffer from obesity can face a number of long-term health problems, including blindness and kidney failure. The trend toward childhood obesity is still increasing, even though there has been an influx of "low-fat," "light" and "fat-free" products on the market. National consumption studies show that people have been eating less total dietary fat over the last couple of decades. So why aren't we getting thinner?

There are a number of reasons, but the root of the problem is that we haven't decreased the total amount of calories consumed; we have only changed the sources of those calories. Instead of high-fat foods, we have switched to highly processed foods full of simple carbohydrates. To manage obesity, North Americans need to make changes in the quantity and quality of the foods they choose. Dieting and exercising alone won't do the trick, because once the diet ends or you are too busy for the gym, the benefits stop. This is where high-fiber foods can muscle in. Foods that are high in fiber, such as whole grains, vegetables and fruits, contribute to a feeling of fullness, or satiety, so that you eat less. Also, insoluble fiber adds no calories; it provides bulk to your meals and so reduces the total calories consumed.

Fiber, Weight Loss and Weight Control

As I stated above, fiber is an important tool in weight loss both for those who just want to shave a few pounds and for those who want to maintain a healthy body weight. Popular commercial diets such as Weight Watchers include fiber as part of their diet plan because they know that high-fiber foods contribute to weight loss by providing low-calorie bulk and eliminating excess fat from your diet. How many people loosen the buttons on their waistbands because they've eaten long after they were full, because that "Stop eating now!" signal from the stomach was delayed? Whole foods take more time to chew, which slows down eating time and gives your body a chance to let you know when it has had enough.

Fiber and Heart Disease

In addition to helping people manage obesity (one of the basic causes of heart disease), fiber can also help control cholesterol levels, thus reducing the risk of heart attack and stroke. Soluble fiber can bind to bile acids that digest fats, moving them through the digestive system. Bile is made from cholesterol, and once eliminated from the body, the liver has to manufacture more to use in the digestion process, by using stored cholesterol. The body, then, uses up harmful excess cholesterol instead of allowing it to roam around damaging your body by forming the plaques that can block arteries and lead to a heart attack or stroke.

Fiber and Diabetes

After a six-year study, the American Medical Association reported that women who ate high-sugar, low-fiber diets (including foods such as white bread and soft drinks) were two and a half times more likely to get diabetes. More and more studies are showing that, regardless of a genetic predisposition to the disease, a healthy lifestyle that includes eating foods high in fiber plays a role in preventing adult-onset diabetes.

In a recent landmark study, the *New England Journal of Medicine* treated patients with Type II diabetes by increasing their fiber intake. They did not take fiber supplements but instead ate fiber-rich foods such as papayas, oranges, grapefruit, sweet potatoes, oat bran, granola, raisins and oatmeal. After the study was over, it was found that both their blood-sugar and cholesterol levels had improved. Similar studies have shown that foods high in soluble fiber can help control or lower blood sugar. This allows the limited insulin system of a person with diabetes to work on converting sugar to energy. Fiber takes longer to digest, so it slows the release of glucose from food into the bloodstream. Increasing the fiber in a patient's diet is similar in effect to taking oral anti-diabetes medication for some people, and can help to prevent the devastating complications of diabetes, which include kidney disease, stroke, heart attack and eye and nerve damage. Of course, fiber is only one piece of the diabetes puzzle; those trying to manage their condition should be under the supervision of medical professionals.

Fiber and Cancer

High-fiber diets have long been linked to the prevention of colon cancer, though there has been much controversy over the effectiveness of high-fiber diets and cancer prevention. Studies that focus only on adding fiber supplements such as bran have failed to show a reduction in cancer risk. Yet studies that focus on whole foods (like those in *Fiber Boost*) that provide both soluble and insoluble fiber have proved more successful. A new European study, the largest ever conducted on nutrition and cancer, involved 500,000 people in ten countries. People were divided into five categories on the basis of dietary-fiber intake; those who ate the most fiber (35 grams a day) had a 40 percent lower risk of colorectal cancer than those who ate the least amount (15 grams a day).

While the exact reason fiber reduces colon-cancer risk is unknown, there are theories. One is that fiber behaves like a bouncer at a nightclub, binding itself to potential cancer-causing compounds and escorting them out of the body, much the same way a bouncer would toss unruly patrons out the door. Another theory is that fiber makes protective changes to the cells, making them more cancer resistant.

The benefits of fiber in preventing cancers that affect the breast, lung, stomach, mouth and esophagus are not as clear. However, there is a definite link between a healthy lifestyle (regular physical activity, maintaining a healthy weight and eating a diet high in naturally fiber-rich foods) and a reduced risk of most cancers.

Diverticular Disease

This is where I have to get into the nitty-gritty of the colon. About half of all North Americans over the age of 60 are affected by diverticulosis, a condition that results in weak spots and small pouches (called diverticula) projecting out of the colon. The pouches are caused by strain and pressure related to irregularity. Unfortunately, most people do not have any early symptoms, which include cramping, bloating or constipation, so the situation is often ignored until more serious complications develop. When the pouches become inflamed, the condition advances and is called diverticulitis. The most common symptoms include abdominal pain, fever, nausea, vomiting, chills, cramping, bleeding and constipation. The dominant theory is that diverticulosis is caused by a low-fiber diet. The disease was first noticed in the United States in the early 1900s, around the same time that processed foods made from refined flour were being introduced into the American diet. Medical professionals know that fiber can help prevent diverticula from forming in the first place and, in most cases, help relieve symptoms.

Gall Bladder Disease

Gallstones are clumps of solid material that form in the gall bladder and can block the duct that carries bile into the digestive system. Gallstones are made up almost entirely of excess cholesterol. The formation of gallstones can result in pain and lead to surgery if the bile duct becomes permanently blocked. Soluble fiber can help prevent the formation of gallstones by ensuring that excess cholesterol is more likely to be eliminated from the body.

Irritable Bowel Syndrome

Irritable bowel syndrome (IBS) is a condition that affects about one in seven people and often plagues sufferers with alternating bouts of constipation and diarrhea, as well as cramping, nausea, bloating and loss of appetite. A low-fat, high-fiber diet can help to manage the symptoms of IBS. Gradually adding fiber, especially soluble fiber, and avoiding other food triggers can help those with IBS to live more comfortably. Those with symptoms should have a thorough checkup by their physicians before changing their diet, to rule out any more serious conditions.

As you can see, eating more fiber on a regular basis can help prevent or manage many of the long-term illnesses that affect the quality of life of millions of North Americans. Old habits are hard to break, and radical changes are rarely maintained. This book is a tool for gradual change and includes many familiar recipes that have been transformed with a healthy twist. It is not a low-fat cookbook but focuses instead on the total nutritional content of the recipe. The emphasis is on reaping all the benefits that wholesome food can provide.

Ten Simple Ways to Increase Fiber Intake

1. Sprinkle wheat and/or oat bran on top of your morning cereal or into smoothies, or use bran instead of breadcrumbs in your burgers and meatballs.
2. Substitute the real thing for your morning juice; eat whole oranges and other fruits instead of just drinking juice.
3. Substitute whole-grain breads and rolls for your usual white-bread versions. Seven- and twelve-grain, pumpernickel, rye and other dense breads have great flavor and require less enhancement with butter, as they are generally moister than white breads.
4. Eat vegetarian one or two nights a week. Try a colorful tofu stir-fry, bean-enhanced salad suppers or hearty minestrone soup.
5. Choose whole-wheat pastas more often for your favorite pasta dishes.
6. Eat legumes frequently; stir into pasta dishes, soups and stews and sprinkle on salads.
7. Eat fresh and frozen berries. Try raspberries on cereal, strawberries in spinach salad or blueberries layered with granola for dessert; they are delicious and nutritious.
8. Substitute whole-wheat flour for white in your baking; in many recipes, up to three-quarters of all-purpose flour can be replaced with whole-wheat flour.
9. Try an appetizing variety of new grains such as brown rice, wild rice, whole-wheat couscous, barley and quinoa in main-course and side dishes.
10. Put vegetables first. Plan menus around the vegetables on your plate at mealtimes instead of starting with the protein and adding vegetables as an afterthought.

Fiber Boosters

Use the following charts to help you choose higher-fiber foods more often.

Very High Sources of Fiber (6 g or more per serving):

Avocado, 1 whole	10.1 g
Barley, 1/2 cup (125 mL), cooked	8.6 g
Beans, baked in tomato sauce, 1/2 cup (125 mL)	7 g
Beans, black, 1/2 cup (125 mL), cooked	6 g
Beans, great northern, 1/2 cup (125 mL), cooked	6.2 g
Beans, lima, 1/2 cup (125 mL), cooked	6.6 g
Beans, navy, 1/2 cup (125 mL), cooked	6.2 g
Blackberries, 1 cup (250 mL)	7.6 g
Bran cereal, 100 %, 1/2 cup (125 mL)	9.9 g
Bulgur, 1/2 cup (125 mL), cooked	9.8 g
Corn, creamed, 1 cup (250 mL)	7.6 g
Cornmeal, 1/2 cup (125 mL)	6.7 g

Dates, 10 dried	7.1 g
Figs, dried, ^{1}/$_2$ cup (125 mL)	12.9 g
Flour, whole-wheat, ^{1}/$_2$ cup (125 mL)	7.6 g
Pasta, whole-wheat, 3 oz (90 g), dry serving	7.1 g
Prunes, 10	6.1 g
Raisins, sultana, 1 cup (250 mL)	6 g
Raspberries, 1 cup (250 mL), frozen	11 g
Raspberries, 1 cup (250 mL), raw	6 g
Seeds, pumpkin, ^{1}/$_2$ cup (50 mL), roasted	7.8 g
Sweet potatoes, 1 cup (250 mL), cooked	8.3 g

High Sources of Fiber (4 g or more per serving):

Apples, dried, 10 rings	5.6 g
Apricots, dried, ^{1}/$_2$ cup (125 mL)	5.4 g
Artichoke, 1 whole, cooked	4.9 g
Beans, kidney, ^{1}/$_2$ cup (125 mL), cooked	5.8 g
Beans, soy, ^{1}/$_2$ cup (125 mL), cooked	4 g
Blueberries, 1 cup (250 mL), frozen	5 g
Blueberries, 1 cup (250 mL), raw	3.8 g
Bread, pumpernickel, 2 slices	4 g
Bread, whole-wheat, 2 slices	4 g
Broccoli, 1 large spear, cooked	4.3 g
English muffin, whole-wheat, 1 whole	4.4 g
Fennel, ^{1}/$_4$ cup (60 mL), raw	5 g
Lentils, ^{1}/$_2$ cup (125 mL), cooked	4.2 g
Oats, large flake, raw, ^{1}/$_2$ cup (125 mL)	5 g
Parsnip, 1 cup (250 mL), cooked	5.8 g
Pear, 1 whole	5.1 g
Pecans, ^{1}/$_2$ cup (125 mL), whole	5.5 g
Pine nuts, ^{1}/$_4$ cup (60 mL)	5.7 g
Pita, whole-wheat, 1 whole	4.7 g
Potato, 1 whole, baked	4.2 g
Quinoa, ^{1}/$_2$ cup (125 mL), cooked	5.9 g
Rhubarb, 1 cup (250 mL), stewed	4.8 g
Rutabaga, 1 cup (250 mL), cooked	4 g
Spinach, ^{1}/$_2$ cup (125 mL), cooked	4.4 g
Textured vegetable protein (TVP), ^{1}/$_4$ cup (60 mL), soaked	4 g
Tomatoes, 1 cup (250 mL), canned	4 g

Sources of Fiber (2 g or more per zserving):

Almonds, unblanched, ^{1}/$_4$ cup (60 mL)	3.5 g
Apple, 1 whole	2.6 g
Applesauce, 1 cup (250 mL)	3.8 g

Banana, 1 whole	2 g
Beans, green, $1/2$ cup (125 mL), cooked	2 g
Beets, $1/2$ cup (125 mL), cooked	2.4 g
Blueberries, 1 cup (250 mL), raw	3.8 g
Bread, rye, dark, 2 slices	3.8 g
Broccoli, 1 large spear, raw	3.6 g
Brown rice, 1 cup (250 mL), cooked	2.8 g
Cabbage, 1 cup (250 mL), cooked	2.8 g
Cabbage, $1/6$ head, raw	2.6 g
Cantaloupe, $1/2$ medium	2.7 g
Carrots, 1 medium, raw	2 g
Carrots, $1/2$ cup (125 mL), cooked	3.2 g
Cherries, sour, 1 cup (250 mL), raw	2.5 g
Chickpeas, $1/2$ cup (125 mL), cooked	3.7 g
Coconut, sweetened, $1/2$ cup (125 mL), shredded	2.4 g
Couscous, $1/2$ cup (125 mL), cooked	2.2 g
Cranberries, $1/2$ cup (125 mL), raw	2.5 g
Fig, 1, whole, fresh	2.1 g
Grapefruit, 1 whole	2.2 g
Grapes, 1 cup (250 mL)	2.2 g
Honeydew melon, $1/4$ medium	2.5 g
Hummus, $1/4$ cup (60 mL)	3.6 g
Kiwi, 1 large	3.1 g
Oatmeal, instant, 48 g pkg ($1^1/2$ oz) cooked with $1/2$ cup (125 mL) boiling water	2.6 g
Okra, $1/2$ cup (125 mL), cooked	2.8 g
Orange, 1 navel	2.3 g
Peanut butter, 2 tbsp (30 mL)	2.2 g
Peanuts, dry-roasted, $1/4$ cup (60 mL)	3.2 g
Pepper, green, 1 whole	2.3 g
Potato, 1 whole, boiled	2.5 g
Pumpkin, $1/2$ cup (125 mL), cooked	3.6 g
Red River cereal, (50 g) serving, prepared (as indicated on box)	2.8 g
Sauerkraut, $1/2$ cup (125 mL)	2.9 g
Seeds, sunflower, $1/4$ cup (60 mL), roasted	3.6 g
Shredded wheat, 1 biscuit	2.4 g
Spinach, 1 cup (250 mL), raw	2.4 g
Squash, summer, 1 cup (250 mL), cooked	3.8 g
Strawberries, 1 cup (250 mL), raw	3.7 g
Tortillas, whole-wheat, 1 10 in (25 cm) wrap	3.6 g
Walnuts, $1/4$ cup (60 mL), whole	2 g

Fiber Boost: Everyday Cooking for a Long, Healthy Life

Healthy Beginnings

A healthy breakfast can be just the right start for accomplishing everything our busy lives throw at us.

Daily Detox Smoothies

All-in-One Muffin Mix

Health-Kick Cereal Bars

Orange-Chocolate Fig Spread

If you have a little more time or are looking for healthful brunch recipes, try:

Multigrain Raspberry Yogurt Parfait

Vanilla Lime-Citrus Starter with Pomegranate

Mix–and-Match Oatmeal Bowls

Whole-Wheat Blueberry Blintzes

Daily Detox Smoothies

PER SERVING	
Calories	157
Fat (g)	1
Protein (g)	2
Carbohydrate (g)	40
Fiber (g)	5
Sodium (mg)	2.5

A high source of fiber. An excellent source of vitamin C and folate.

Serves 2

Detoxify every day with this delicious meal in a glass. With a boost of fiber and vitamin C, it is perfectly portable for those on the run. The key to a thick, creamy shake is frozen bananas, so keep a container of banana chunks in your freezer just for this purpose.

1/2 cup	frozen cranberries	125 mL
1 cup	cubed frozen banana	250 mL
1 cup	unsweetened orange juice	250 mL
2 tbsp	natural wheat bran	30 mL

Combine the frozen cranberries, banana, orange juice and wheat bran in a blender. Blend until smooth.

TIP: For more protein, substitute plain or vanilla soy milk or yogurt for half the orange juice.

Breakfast in a Blender

Smoothies are becoming the trend for the health-conscious. Blender bars are popping up on urban street corners for those who want a quick meal replacement, energy boost or healthful detox. Got a busy schedule? Smoothies can be whizzed up and taken on the road. Pack your freezer with cubes of bananas, and a variety of berries and other frozen fruit to be blended with juice, soy milk or yogurt for a wholesome shake. Sprinkle in a little wheat bran for extra fiber—you'll hardly notice it!

All-in-One Muffin Mix

Makes 12 large muffins

Fresh from the oven, muffins are a tasty breakfast treat or midday snack. Personalize the basic mix to suit your family by choosing your favorite flavor variations below.

¹/₂ cup	all-purpose flour	125 mL
¹/₂ cup	whole-wheat flour	125 mL
¹/₂ cup	rolled oats, large flakes	125 mL
¹/₂ cup	natural wheat bran	125 mL
²/₃ cup	brown sugar	150 mL
1 tbsp	baking powder	15 mL
2	large eggs	2
1 cup	buttermilk	250 mL
¹/₂ cup	vegetable oil	125 mL

Preheat the oven to 375°F (190°C). Stir the all-purpose flour, whole-wheat flour, oats, bran, brown sugar and baking powder in a large bowl until combined. In a separate bowl, whisk the eggs, buttermilk and oil until combined.

Make a well in the center of the dry ingredients and pour in the wet ingredients. Use a wooden spoon or spatula to stir just until combined. Spoon into 12 greased or paper-lined muffin tins. Bake in the preheated oven for 20 to 25 minutes or until the tops spring back when gently touched.

Variations:
Orange Date: Stir 1 cup (250 mL) chopped dates into the dry mixture and 1 tbsp (15 mL) finely grated orange rind into the wet mixture.

Cranberry Lemon: Stir 1 cup (250 mL) dried cranberries into the dry mixture and 1 tbsp (15 mL) finely grated lemon rind into the wet mixture. Drizzle the finished muffins with a combination of ¹/₂ cup (125 mL) icing sugar and 1 tbsp (15 mL) lemon juice.

Apple Cheddar: Stir 1 cup (250 mL) chopped dried apples, ¹/₂ cup (125 mL) shredded old cheddar cheese and 1 tbsp (15 mL) ground cinnamon into the dry mixture.

Recipe Makeover: This recipe includes whole wheat, oatmeal, bran and dried fruit. It provides both a soluble and insoluble fiber boost to typically calorie-laden muffins.

ORANGE DATE
PER SERVING

Calories	287
Fat (g)	11
Protein (g)	5
Carbohydrate (g)	46
Fiber (g)	5
Sodium (mg)	122

A high source of fiber. An excellent source of vitamin D.

CRANBERRY LEMON
PER SERVING

Calories	276
Fat (g)	11
Protein (g)	5
Carbohydrate (g)	43
Fiber (g)	4
Sodium (mg)	123

A high source of fiber. An excellent source of vitamin D.

APPLE CHEDDAR
PER SERVING

Calories	389
Fat (g)	14
Protein (g)	8
Carbohydrate (g)	63
Fiber (g)	7
Sodium (mg)	232

A very high source of fiber. An excellent source of vitamin D.

Health-Kick Cereal Bars

PER SERVING	
Calories	286
Fat (g)	13
Protein (g)	7
Carbohydrate (g)	41
Fiber (g)	4
Sodium (mg)	61
A high source of fiber.	

Makes 12 bars

Breakfast to go, with the classic flavors of peanut butter and banana to appeal to adults and kids alike.

1 cup	light peanut butter	250 mL
1/2 cup	brown sugar	125 mL
1/2 cup	liquid honey	125 mL
1 cup	instant or quick-cooking oats	250 mL
3 cups	raisin bran–style cereal	750 mL
3/4 cup	chopped dried bananas (or banana chips)	175 mL
2 tbsp	ground flax seeds	30 mL

Combine the peanut butter, brown sugar and honey in a heavy saucepan set over medium heat. Bring to the boil, stirring constantly. In a large bowl, combine the oats, cereal, bananas and flax seeds. Pour the hot peanut-butter mixture over the cereal and stir until the cereal is well coated. Press the mixture into a greased 8-inch (2 L) square baking pan. Chill until firm.

Cereal Selection

Many of the breakfast cereals available on supermarket shelves are full of refined flour and sugar. When shopping, read the labels and choose cereals with whole grains instead of the less nutritious fad cereals. Check out the Fiber Boosters charts on page 9–11 for ideas.

Orange-Chocolate Fig Spread

Makes 1 cup (250 mL)

Instead of simply grabbing butter or jam, spread this exotic breakfast treat on your toast. Its orange and chocolate flavors will appeal to young and old alike, and the figs add a fiber boost as well as other nutrients.

1 cup	chopped dried figs, about 12	250 mL
1/2 cup	softened butter or non-hydrogenated margarine	125 mL
3 tbsp	unsweetened cocoa powder	45 mL
2 tbsp	brown sugar	30 mL
1 tbsp	finely grated orange peel	15 mL

Combine the figs, butter, cocoa, brown sugar and orange peel in a food processor and process until smooth. Let stand at least 15 minutes before using. Pack into a crock, cover and refrigerate for up to 5 days.

TIP: Serve this delicious spread on dried apple slices as an after-school or at-work snack.

Fabulous Figs

Figs were considered a sacred fruit by ancient peoples and were thought to be a symbol of peace and prosperity. Ranging in color from purple to white, their somewhat pear-shaped skins contain a multitude of fibrous edible seeds. Fresh figs, in season from June to October, are extremely perishable and should be used soon after buying, within two or three days. Dried figs are available year-round and can be used like any dried fruit. Figs are a good source of iron, calcium and phosphorus as well as fiber.

PER SERVING (2 tbsp/ 30 mL)	
Calories	183
Fat (g)	12
Protein (g)	1
Carbohydrate (g)	21
Fiber (g)	4
Sodium (mg)	120

A high source of fiber.

Recipe Makeover:
Delicious figs add a fiber boost to this, which you can use on your breakfast breads instead of butter or cream cheese.

Multigrain Raspberry Yogurt Parfait

PER SERVING	
Calories	302
Fat (g)	7
Protein (g)	12
Carbohydrate (g)	48
Fiber (g)	6
Sodium (mg)	142

A very high source of fiber. An excellent source of vitamin B_{12} and calcium.

Makes 4 parfaits

Grain-enhanced yogurt is becoming a trendy health-food snack. This fiber-rich breakfast capitalizes on a delicious way to eat whole grains.

2 tbsp	Red River-style cereal*	30 mL
1/2 cup	water	125 mL
3 cups	vanilla yogurt or your favorite flavor	750 mL
2 cups	raspberries, fresh or unsweetened frozen, thawed	500 mL
1 cup	granola (recipe in Mixed Berry Crunch Trifle, page 118, or commercial)	250 mL

Combine the Red River cereal and water in a pan set over medium-high heat, and bring to a boil. Reduce the heat and simmer for 4 minutes or until most of the water is absorbed. Cool to room temperature. Blend the cooked cereal with the yogurt.

Divide half the raspberries among 4 parfait glasses. Top with half the yogurt mixture. Repeat the layers. Top the parfaits with the granola.

*Red River cereal is a whole-grain cereal that contains cracked wheat, rye and flax. It contains 5.7 g of fiber per cooked serving. If it is unavailable, substitute 1/2 cup (125 mL) cooked mixed whole grains.

TIP: Look for yogurt that contains both acidophilus and bifidum cultures, which promote healthy intestinal flora.

TIP: You can substitute blueberries or blackberries for the raspberries.

Vanilla Lime-Citrus Starter with Pomegranate

Serves 4

This refreshing sweet-and-tart salad will give you a morning boost. Pomegranate seeds add an interesting crunch as well as visual appeal, but you can substitute dried berries instead.

1/4 cup	granulated sugar	60 mL
1/4 cup	water	60 mL
2 tbsp	fresh lime juice	30 mL
1	vanilla bean or 1 tsp (5 mL) pure vanilla extract	1
2	red grapefruits	2
2	large navel oranges	2
1 tsp	finely grated lime peel	5 mL
2 tbsp	pomegranate seeds	30 mL

PER SERVING	
Calories	128
Fat (g)	0
Protein (g)	1
Carbohydrate (g)	32
Fiber (g)	2
Sodium (mg)	1

A source of fiber. An excellent source of vitamin C.

Combine the sugar, water and lime juice in a small saucepan set over medium heat. Split the vanilla bean in half lengthwise and add to saucepan. Bring the mixture to a boil, stirring until the sugar dissolves. Reduce the heat to low and simmer for 1 minute. Pull out the vanilla bean halves and cool until they are easy to handle. Run a butter knife along the cut sides and scrape the seeds into the syrup. Chill the syrup. (The syrup can be made ahead and kept in a sealed jar in the refrigerator for up to 1 week.)

Use a sharp knife to cut the peel off the grapefruit and the oranges, being careful to remove all the bitter pith (the white portion below the skin). Slice the fruit, removing any visible seeds. Toss with chilled syrup and lime peel. Serve immediately in cocktail dishes garnished with pomegranate seeds.

A Good Start

For optimum nutrition, eat whole citrus fruits instead of drinking fruit juice. Juices provide less fiber and typically more calories (in the form of added sugars) than the whole fruit. Eating whole fruits will also make you feel fuller longer, and you will be less likely to crave snacks between meals.

Mix-and-Match Oatmeal Bowls

PER SERVING (topped with nuts and fruit)	
Calories	119
Fat (g)	3
Protein (g)	4
Carbohydrate (g)	20
Fiber (g)	3
Sodium (mg)	3
A source of fiber.	

Serves 4 (doubles easily)

Instead of frying up bacon and eggs for your next family brunch, stir up a large batch of oatmeal and arrange a buffet of toppings. People can add their own favorite flavors to the bowl. Serve muffins and fresh fruit on the side.

3 cups	water	750 mL
1/2 tsp	salt (or to taste)	2 mL
1 1/2 cups	rolled oats (instant, quick-cooking or large flake old-fashioned)	375 mL

Bring the water and salt to the boil in a large saucepan. Add the oats and bring mixture back to the boil. Reduce heat and simmer, stirring occasionally, until thickened slightly, about 3 to 5 minutes. Remove the pot from the heat, cover, and let stand for 3 minutes before serving.

Suggested Oatmeal Toppings:
- Milk, light cream or yogurt
- Dried fruit
- Low-sugar jams
- Maple and fruit syrups
- Fresh or frozen thawed berries
- Diced apple
- Granola
- Toasted nuts
- Flax seeds
- Spiced sugars such as cinnamon sugar or ginger sugar

A fun idea: Make up cards for the buffet table with oatmeal recipe ideas to make it fun for adults and kids alike. Here are a couple of suggestions to get you started:

Apple Pie
Combine 2 tsp (10 mL) granulated sugar with 1/4 tsp (1 mL) ground cinnamon. Stir into the oatmeal along with 1/4 cup (60 mL) chopped dried apple. Serve with a sprinkle of sharp cheddar cheese.

Berries and Cream
Stir 1/4 cup (60 mL) vanilla yogurt into the oatmeal along with 1 tbsp (15 mL) strawberry jam.

Whole-Wheat Blueberry Blintzes

Makes about 12 blintzes

A festive dish featuring wild blueberries, light cottage cheese, a tender whole-wheat crêpe and a caramel orange sauce. It's so delicious, you'll forget it is good for you.

Crêpes:

1/2 cup	whole-wheat flour	125 mL
1/2 cup	all-purpose flour	125 mL
1 cup	milk	250 mL
3/4 cup	water	175 mL
3	eggs	3
2 tbsp	granulated sugar	30 mL
1/4 tsp	salt	1 mL
1 tbsp	each melted butter and vegetable oil, combined	15 mL

Blueberry Cheese Filling:

1 cup	frozen wild blueberries, thawed	250 mL
2	packages (each 8 oz/250 g) pressed cottage cheese	2
3 tbsp	granulated sugar	45 mL
1 tbsp	orange liqueur or fresh orange juice	15 mL
1 tbsp	finely grated orange peel	15 mL

Caramel Orange Sauce:

1 cup	granulated sugar	250 mL
1/4 cup	water	60 mL
1/3 cup	fresh orange juice	75 mL
1/4 cup	sliced almonds, toasted (see Tip, page 40)	60 mL

Crêpes:

Combine flours with milk, water, eggs, sugar and salt in a blender or in a large bowl, using a whisk. Blend until smooth, scraping down the sides once, for about 1 minute. Let stand at room temperature for 1 hour or for up to 24 hours in the refrigerator.

Heat a medium nonstick or crêpe pan over medium heat. Brush the pan with a little of the butter and oil mixture. Stir the batter and spoon 3 tbsp (45 mL) into the center of the pan; swirl the pan to coat it evenly. Cook for 1 to 2 minutes or until the top is set and the bottom golden. Use a thin spatula to flip the crêpe and quickly brown the second side. Repeat with the remaining batter, greasing the pan as needed, to make about 12 crêpes. Layer them between sheets of waxed paper until ready to fill.

Recipe Makeover: Adding whole-wheat flour to the crêpe batter gives this brunch dish a fiber boost.

Blueberry Cheese Filling:

Drain blueberries well. Fold into the cheese along with the sugar, orange liqueur and orange peel. Reserve.

Caramel Orange Sauce:

In a deep, heavy-bottomed saucepan, stir sugar into the water. Set pan over medium heat and cook without stirring until a clear syrup forms and the sugar is dissolved. Increase the heat to high, and bring the syrup to a rolling boil. Boil, without stirring, until the syrup becomes an amber color. Remove the pan from the heat, and, standing back, carefully pour in the orange juice. (The mixture will sputter and spit, so be careful.) Stir the sauce until smooth. Serve at once or let cool to room temperature.

To assemble the blintzes:

Preheat the oven to 325°F (160°C). Lay a crêpe on a clean work surface and spoon ¼ cup (50 mL) of the cheese mixture into the center. Fold over the corners to make a square package and lay seam side down in a greased 9- × 13-inch (3 L) baking dish. Repeat with the remaining crêpes and drizzle with the caramel sauce. Sprinkle with toasted almonds. Cover tightly with foil and place in the preheated oven. Bake for 20 minutes or until warmed through.

TIP: Cover your hand with a towel or oven mitt when adding the orange juice to the syrup.

Singing the Blues

Frozen wild blueberries should be a freezer staple. They contain more fiber per cup than fresh and can be tossed into smoothies, fruit salads, pies, muffins and more.

Great for Grazing

Whether you're hosting a small get-together or toting a potluck dish, it is often hard to come up with healthful appetizer ideas. Here's a sample of recipes that you don't have to feel guilty about snacking on:

Smoky Chipotle Pepper Dip

Whole-Wheat Mini Calzones

Maple-Stout Meatballs

Buckwheat Blinis with Avocado Salsa

Sun-Dried Tomato and Goat Cheese Baguette Bites

Gorgonzola-Stuffed Dates

Take It Away—Quick Sandwich Solutions

Smoky Chipotle Pepper Dip

Makes approximately 2½ cups (625 mL)

PER SERVING (4 tsp/ 20 mL)	
Calories	60
Fat (g)	2
Protein (g)	2
Carbohydrate (g)	10
Fiber (g)	2
Sodium (mg)	186

A source of fiber. An excellent source of vitamin A.

A favorite of all who try it, this low-fat dip is delicious scooped up on whole-wheat pita wedges. Chipotle peppers are sold in cans and have a wonderful smoky heat. If canned chipotles are unavailable in your area, add your favorite hot pepper sauce to taste.

2	red peppers, cored and halved	2
1	can (19 oz/540 mL) chickpeas, drained and rinsed	1
2	canned chipotle peppers with sauce	2
2 tbsp	lemon juice	30 mL
2 tbsp	minced onion	30 mL
1	clove garlic, minced	1
1 tbsp	olive oil	15 mL
1 tbsp	red wine vinegar	15 mL
½ tsp	each salt and freshly ground pepper	2 mL

Preheat a grill to medium-high. Place the red pepper halves on the grill. Grill, turning as needed, until well marked and tender, about 10 minutes. Remove from grill and place immediately into a paper bag to loosen the skins. Using your fingers, peel the peppers and discard skins.

Combine the peppers, chickpeas, chipotle peppers, lemon juice, onion, garlic, olive oil and vinegar in a food processor or blender and purée until smooth. (If you are using a blender, you may need to add up to 2 tbsp/ 30 mL water to help the mixture blend.) Taste and season the dip with salt and pepper as desired. Transfer the mixture to a serving bowl or airtight container and refrigerate for at least 1 hour before serving to meld the flavors. Serve with crudités such as carrot and celery sticks and crackers.

TIP: You can substitute 4 roasted red peppers from a jar or oven-roast fresh peppers instead of grilling: Preheat the oven to 350°F (180°C). Set the halves in the oven (right on the rack), skin-side-down. Roast for 20 to 30 minutes, turning once, until the skins are well charred and the peppers are softened. Proceed as above.

"Dip"endable

Puréed chickpeas give this dip body and flavor while decreasing the fat content and providing a fiber boost. Beans are also budget-friendly, something to keep in mind when entertaining. Try substituting some puréed legumes (such as chickpeas or navy beans) for the higher-fat sour cream, cream cheese or mayonnaise in your favorite dip recipes.

Whole-Wheat Mini Calzones

Makes 16 calzones

This basic dough recipe can be used as the base for your favorite pizza toppings as well. Choose from the gourmet fillings on the next page or create your own combinations. The mini calzones are freezable and make an excellent appetizer, snack or lunch option.

Dough:

2¼ cups	whole-wheat flour	550 mL
1 cup	all-purpose flour (approx.)	250 mL
2	packages (each ¼ oz/7 g) quick-rising yeast	2
1½ tsp	salt	7 mL
1 tbsp	honey	15 mL
1½ cups	very hot water	375 mL
1 tbsp	olive oil (approx.)	15 mL
½ cup	cornmeal	125 mL

Combine the whole-wheat flour with the all-purpose flour, yeast, salt and honey in a large bowl. Add the hot water and olive oil and stir with a fork until the mixture makes a ragged dough. Turn out onto a lightly floured board and knead for 5 minutes or until smooth and elastic, adding up to ¼ cup (50 mL) more flour as needed. Form the dough into a ball and transfer to a bowl greased with oil, turning to coat the dough. Cover with a damp tea towel and let stand in a warm, draft-free area for 15 minutes.

To make the calzones:
Divide the dough into 16 equal pieces and press or roll each one into a 4-inch (10 cm) circle. Place 2 tbsp (15 mL) of your choice of filling (see page 26) in the center. Use your fingertip to wet the outer edge of the circle and fold over, pressing to seal the edges. Prick the calzone with a fork, then press each side gently into the cornmeal. Set on a greased baking sheet. (Calzones can be frozen at this point and stored in an airtight container between layers of cornmeal-topped waxed paper for up to 1 month.)

Preheat the oven to 400°F (200°C) and bake the calzones on a cookie sheet for about 10 minutes or until golden all over (add 5 to 7 minutes if frozen). Serve warm.

Gourmet Fillings

Balsamic Mushroom Filling:

1 tbsp	olive oil	15 mL
1	small onion, sliced	1
1	clove garlic, minced	1
8 oz	mixed wild mushrooms, chopped roughly	250 g
1 tbsp	balsamic vinegar	15 mL
1/2 tsp	each salt and freshly ground pepper	2 mL
2 tbsp	chopped fresh basil	15 mL
4 oz	provolone or mozzarella cheese, shredded	125 g

Heat the oil in a nonstick pan set over medium heat. Add the onion and cook until golden, about 8 minutes. Stir in the garlic and mushrooms and cook until lightly browned. Stir in the vinegar, salt and pepper and cook until the liquid is absorbed. Stir in the basil and cool to room temperature. Stir in the cheese and reserve.

Grilled Eggplant and Feta Filling:

1	small eggplant, about 3/4 lb (350 g)	1
1 tbsp	olive oil	15 mL
1/2 tsp	dried oregano	2 mL
1/2 tsp	each salt and freshly ground pepper	2 mL
2 tbsp	sun-dried tomato paste or very finely chopped sun-dried tomatoes	30 mL
1/2 cup	crumbled feta or Parmesan cheese	125 mL

Recipe Makeover: The whole wheat gives a fiber boost to this versatile recipe.

Preheat the grill to medium. Thinly slice eggplant into lengths or rounds. Combine olive oil with oregano and brush over slices. Sprinkle eggplant with salt and pepper and lay on the preheated grate. Grill for 6 to 8 minutes or until well marked and tender, turning as needed. Cool the eggplant slightly and chop roughly. Combine with the sun-dried tomato paste or chopped sun-dried tomatoes and cheese and reserve.

Pizza Party!

To use the dough as a pizza base, divide into 2 portions and roll each into a 12-inch (30 cm) round. Top with your favorite topping, such as pizza sauce, sliced pepperoni, mushrooms, peppers, pineapple and cheese, then bake in the lower third of a 400°F (200°C) oven for 10 to 15 minutes, until the bottom is crispy and the cheese is bubbly and golden.

Maple-Stout Meatballs

Makes about 20 meatballs

Because of the secret ingredient, soy, these meatballs are lower in fat than traditional meatballs, but they still have that essential beefy flavor. Serve these winners at your next kick-off party!

PER SERVING (4 meatballs)	
Calories	393
Fat (g)	12
Protein (g)	39
Carbohydrate (g)	34
Fiber (g)	3
Sodium (mg)	1085

A source of fiber. An excellent source of vitamin D, folate, iron, phosphorus and zinc.

Sauce:

1 cup	stout beer or ginger ale	250 mL
1 cup	ketchup	250 mL
1/3 cup	maple syrup	75 mL
2 tbsp	Dijon mustard	30 mL
1 tbsp	lime juice	15 mL

Meatballs:

1 cup	TVP (textured vegetable protein)	250 mL
3/4 cup	hot beef broth	175 mL
1	egg	1
1/4 cup	minced onion	60 mL
1/4 cup	fresh whole-wheat breadcrumbs	60 mL
2	cloves garlic, chopped	2
1 tsp	dry mustard	5 mL
1/2 tsp	each salt and freshly ground pepper	2 mL
3/4 lb	lean ground beef	350 g

Preheat the oven to 350°F (180°C). Stir the stout with the ketchup, maple syrup, Dijon mustard and lime juice in a large bowl and reserve.

Soak the TVP in the beef broth for 15 minutes. In a medium bowl, whisk the egg with the onion, breadcrumbs, garlic, dry mustard, salt and pepper. Crumble in the ground beef and the hydrated TVP. With your hands, gently mix until well combined, then shape into 2-inch (5 cm) balls, about 20.

Set the meatballs on a foil-lined baking sheet and bake in the preheated oven for 20 minutes or until cooked through. Transfer to a deep casserole and pour the reserved sauce over top. Bake, uncovered, for 30 minutes or until heated through, stirring gently occasionally.

TIP: Make a double batch and put the extra meatballs in the freezer to toss into hearty soups or add to tomato sauce for spaghetti (whole-wheat noodles, of course) and meatballs. At parties, keep meatballs hot by serving them from a crockpot set on low. Have toothpicks or small wooden skewers on the side for easy nibbling.

Recipe Makeover:
Traditional meatballs get a fiber boost if you replace half the beef with TVP.

TVP Tips

TVP (textured vegetable protein) is a meat alternative made from soy flour that is formed into granules to add "meaty" bulk to vegetarian dishes. You can find it sold dry in the bulk- or health-food sections of your grocery store. Ready-to-use, pre-seasoned versions of TVP can also be found in the produce section of the grocery store. Many of your favorite foods have a TVP alternative, including chicken fingers, meatballs and burgers. Dry TVP can be stored in your pantry and rehydrated easily with equal parts boiling water or broth. Because it doesn't need browning like meat, it can be tossed into casseroles, stews and pasta dishes and just heated through quickly. TVP is low in fat and a good source of iron and folate.

Buckwheat Blinis with Avocado Salsa

Makes 30 blinis

Traditionally, these little Russian pancakes are made of a light yeast buckwheat dough and served with sour cream and caviar. This Mexican twist makes delightful little appetizers topped with a vibrant green avocado salsa.

Blinis:

2 tsp	quick-rising yeast	10 mL
1 tbsp	honey	15 mL
3/4 cup	warm water	175 mL
1 cup	buckwheat flour	250 mL
1/4 cup	melted butter	60 mL
2 tbsp	sour cream	30 mL
2	large eggs, separated	2
1/4 tsp	salt	1 mL

Avocado Salsa:

2	avocados, peeled and diced	2
2	tomatoes, seeded and diced	2
1	jalapeño pepper, seeded and diced	1
1/4 cup	finely chopped cilantro	60 mL
1 tsp	finely grated lime peel	5 mL
2 tbsp	lime juice	30 mL
1 tsp	each salt and freshly ground pepper	5 mL
1/2 cup	sour cream (optional)	125 mL
	Cilantro leaves (optional)	

Stir the yeast with the honey and warm water. Let mixture stand for 5 minutes or until foamy. Stir in the flour, half the melted butter, sour cream and egg yolks until smooth. Cover the bowl with plastic wrap and let the batter stand for 30 minutes. In a clean bowl, beat the egg whites with the salt until stiff peaks form. Gently fold the egg whites thoroughly into the rest of the batter.

Preheat a large nonstick skillet over medium-high heat and brush with some of the remaining butter. Working in batches, spoon the batter into the skillet in heaping tablespoonfuls to make coin-sized blinis. Cook just until bubbles form on the surface of the blinis. Turn the blinis with a thin, flexible spatula, and cook until lightly browned on the bottom. Repeat with the remaining batter, brushing the pan with more melted butter as needed. Transfer the blinis to a covered tray and set in a warm oven until ready to serve.

Avocado Salsa:

In a small bowl, combine the avocados, tomatoes, jalapeño, cilantro, lime peel, lime juice, salt and pepper. Gently toss until combined. Taste and adjust seasonings, adding more salt if needed.

To serve the blinis:

Place warm pancakes on a platter and top each one with a dollop of the salsa. Garnish with a little sour cream and cilantro leaves if desired.

Buckwheat Bio

Buckwheat is often thought of as a cereal, but it is actually an herb. Buckwheat flour has a pleasant nutty flavor and can be added to baked goods, but it is commonly found in this Russian pancake recipe and in Asian soba noodles. Buckwheat flour can be purchased in bulk- or health-food stores.

Photo: Mix-and-Match Oatmeal Bowls (page 22)

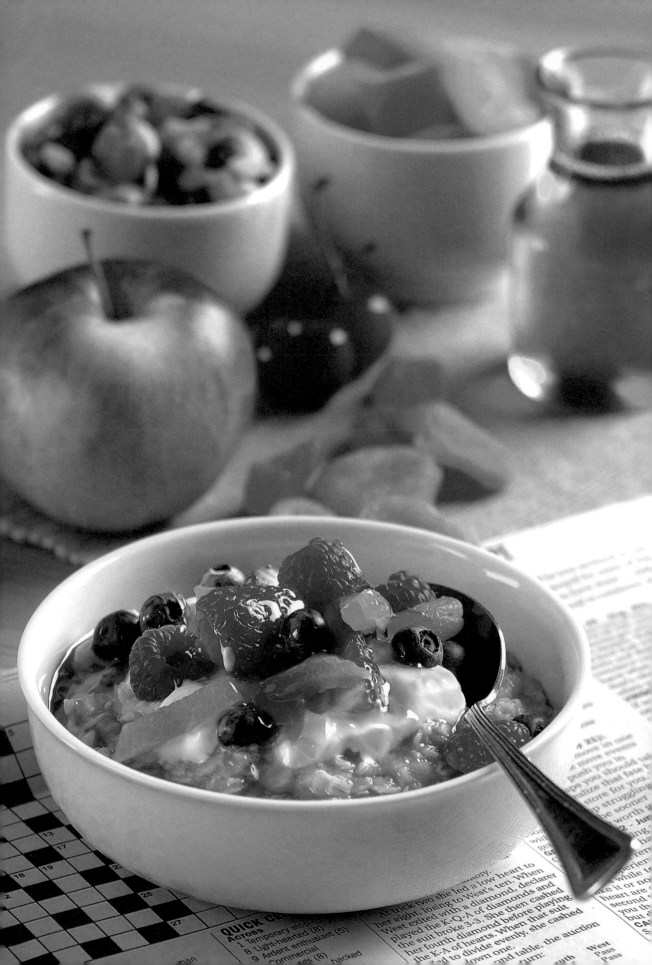

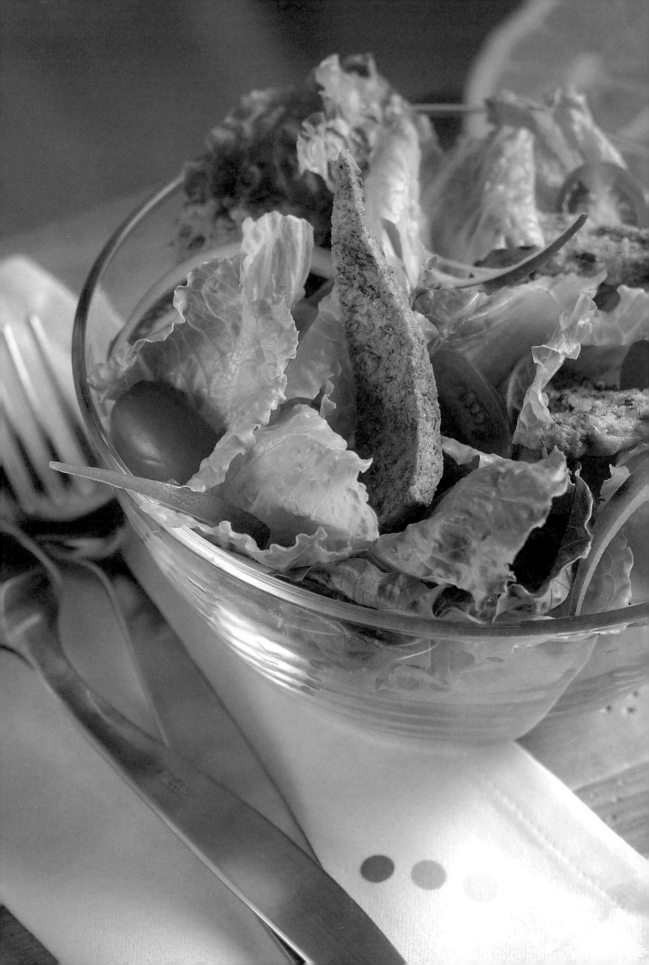

Sun-Dried Tomato and Goat Cheese Baguette Bites

Makes 24 pieces

A pretty and very speedy starter, these can be prepared ahead and simply sliced when the guests arrive. Instead of using a baguette, the filling can be spread over whole-wheat tortillas and rolled to make pinwheel-style appetizers as well.

1	whole-wheat baguette, about 20 inches (50 cm) long	1
½ cup	oil-packed sun-dried tomatoes, about 10 halves	125 mL
¼ cup	lightly packed basil leaves	60 mL
8 oz	creamy goat cheese	250 g
4 oz	softened brick-style light cream cheese	125 g
¼ cup	toasted pine nuts	60 mL
¼ tsp	freshly ground pepper	1 mL

Slice the baguette in half lengthwise with a serrated knife, and remove the bread from the center of each half, leaving a ½-inch- (1 cm) thick shell. (Freeze the extra bread for another use.) Reserve.

Drain the tomatoes and lay out on paper towels to absorb the excess oil. Use a pair of clean, sharp kitchen scissors or a chef's knife to finely sliver the tomatoes and basil. Blend goat cheese with the cream cheese, pine nuts, tomatoes and basil. Stuff the filling into the hollowed-out halves of the baguette, then put the halves together to make a complete loaf. Wrap the loaf in plastic wrap and refrigerate for at least 1 hour or for up to 24 hours. Slice into 1-inch (2.5 cm) rounds to serve.

Photo: Hummus Salad (page 40)

Gorgonzola-Stuffed Dates

PER SERVING (1 date)	
Calories	254
Fat (g)	3
Protein (g)	3
Carbohydrate (g)	61
Fiber (g)	7
Sodium (mg)	49
A very high source of fiber.	

Makes 24 appetizers

Nippy Gorgonzola cheese is an excellent foil for sweet dates, and together they make a simple yet elegant appetizer. For best results, try to find plump Medjool dates.

4 oz	light cream cheese	125 g
2 oz	Gorgonzola cheese	60 g
2 tsp	finely grated orange peel	10 mL
1 tsp	maple syrup	5 mL
24	whole pitted dates	24

Preheat the broiler to high. Process the cream cheese with the Gorgonzola, orange peel and maple syrup in a food processor until smooth. Pipe or spoon the cheese mixture into the dates. Arrange the dates on a parchment-lined cookie sheet and broil for 1 to 2 minutes per side or until browned and warmed through.

It's a Date

Native to the Middle East, dates are grown in hot, dry climates. The oval fruits are green when unripe and, when dried, have a wrinkly appearance. About 1 to 2 inches (2.5 to 5 cm) long, they have a long seed that must be removed before eating. The best-quality dates for stuffing are the jumbo Medjool variety sold in boxes in the produce section of the supermarket. You can also buy pitted dates sold in blocks or chopped in the bulk-food section. They are delicious eaten whole, and they add wonderful sweetness to baked goods.

Take It Away—Quick Sandwich Solutions

Boost the nutritional quotient and add variety to your sandwiches with the following appetizing ideas. Eat the sandwiches right away or wrap tightly in plastic wrap and store in the refrigerator or in a cooler bag until ready to eat.

Garden Veggie Wraps:

Spread a large whole-wheat tortilla with 2 tbsp (30 mL) light cream cheese blended with light ranch dressing. Sprinkle with ½ cup (125 mL) chopped vegetables such as broccoli, celery, carrot, cucumber, sweet pepper and onion. Top with ¼ cup (50 mL) shredded cheddar cheese, and roll up tightly. Makes 1 wrap.

Curried Tuna and Couscous Pita:

Blend ½ cup (125 mL) cooked whole-wheat couscous with 1 can (16 oz/170 g) flaked tuna, 1 diced Granny Smith apple, 2 tbsp (30 mL) mayonnaise, 1 tsp (5 mL) lime juice and ½ tsp (2 mL) curry paste. Stuff the mixture into 2 lettuce-lined whole-wheat pitas. Makes 2 pita sandwiches.

Grilled Vegetables and Mozzarella on a Bun:

Spread a toasted whole-wheat crusty roll with Smoky Chipotle Pepper Dip (page 24), and top with grilled vegetables such as sliced zucchini, eggplant or portobello mushrooms. Top with sliced tomatoes and mozzarella cheese. Serve warm or cold. Makes 1 sandwich.

Avocado and Cucumber on Pumpernickel:

Top a toasted and halved pumpernickel bagel with slices of cucumber and avocado. Drizzle with honey mustard. Serve immediately. Makes 1 open-faced sandwich.

Ham and Pineapple Mini Pizzas:

Top each half of toasted (whole-wheat) English muffins with a spoonful of tomato sauce, a slice of ham, a ring of pineapple and a slice of mozzarella or cheddar cheese. Broil briefly before serving. Makes 2 mini pizzas.

Dressed-for-Success Salads

Salads are the staple of the diet-conscious and an excellent way to increase the veggie content of your daily menu. A salad makes a great side dish, main course, buffet option or light lunch.

Wilted Spinach Salad with Grapefruit and Avocado

Hummus Salad

Mango Tango Slaw

Diva Pasta Salad

Indian Princess Salad

Auckland Chicken Salad

Southwestern Supper Salad

Wilted Spinach Salad with Grapefruit and Avocado

PER SERVING	
Calories	141
Fat (g)	11
Protein (g)	4
Carbohydrate (g)	11
Fiber (g)	4
Sodium (mg)	80

A high source of fiber. An excellent source of vitamin A, folate and magnesium.

Serves 6

Sweet, savory, tangy and salty flavors are combined in this vibrant salad, which is best served immediately after tossing, when the avocado is still brilliant green and the spinach is slightly warm.

1	small red onion	1
1	grapefruit	1
8 cups	baby spinach leaves	2 L
2 tbsp	vegetable oil	30 mL
1	slice bacon, chopped	1
1	clove garlic, minced	1
1 tbsp	maple syrup	15 mL
1/4 tsp	salt	1 mL
1 tbsp	white wine vinegar	15 mL
1	avocado	1
	Freshly ground pepper to taste	

Slice the red onion thinly; mince enough to make 2 tbsp (30 mL) for the dressing; reserve the remaining slices for the salad. Finely grate enough grapefruit peel to make 1 tsp (5 mL), then remove the remaining skin and cut the fruit into segments. Wash and dry spinach and place in a large salad bowl before preparing the dressing.

Heat the oil in a small nonstick skillet set over medium heat, add bacon and cook until crispy. Strain out the bacon bits and drain on paper towels, leaving the oil in the pan. Reduce the heat to medium-low. Stir in the minced onion and garlic and cook just until soft. Add the maple syrup and salt and stir until bubbly. Remove the pan from heat and stir in the vinegar and grapefruit peel. Keep the dressing hot by holding on the cooling element or warming in the microwave.

Cut the avocado in half, remove the pit and, with a sharp knife, score the flesh lengthwise and crosswise. Use a spoon to remove the cubes of avocado from the skin. Toss the avocado cubes with the grapefruit pieces to keep them from browning.

Pour the hot dressing over the spinach and toss until the greens are slightly wilted. Arrange mixture on 6 salad plates and top with onion slices, grapefruit and avocado. Sprinkle with the reserved bacon bits.

The Scoop on Avocados

Avocados are a nutritional wonder. One half of an avocado contains 5 grams of fiber making it a delicious high source. This vibrant, green fruit also contains vitamins E and B_6, which are essential for a healthy immune system and help to prevent hardening of the arteries. Beyond guacamole, avocados can be sliced into salads, sandwiches and fresh salsas. Choose avocados that yield to gentle pressure, or ripen harder avocados overnight by putting them in a paper bag with a ripe banana. Avocado flesh browns quickly when exposed to air. Brushing or tossing with lemon or lime juice will help to preserve the brilliant color.

Hummus Salad

Makes 4 main-course or 8 side-dish servings

This makeover version of a classic Caesar combines the garlicky goodness of hummus with crispy toasted pitas and crunchy romaine lettuce. The dressing can be assembled quickly with store-bought hummus, but you can substitute your own favorite recipe or the one below.

1/3 cup	hummus	75 mL
1 tbsp	lemon juice	15 mL
4 tbsp	extra-virgin olive oil, divided	60 mL
1/4 tsp	freshly ground coarse black pepper	1 mL
2	whole-wheat pitas	2
1/2 tsp	paprika	2 mL
1/4 tsp	salt	1 mL
1	clove garlic, halved	1
8 cups	torn romaine lettuce	2 L
1 cup	thinly sliced red onion	250 mL
1 cup	grape tomatoes, halved	250 mL
	Lemon wedges	

Recipe Makeover: This Caesar-inspired salad reduces the fat content while delivering a fiber boost with a garlicky bean dressing and whole-wheat pita croutons. Add even more fiber and a bacon-like twist by substituting 1/4 cup (60 mL) chopped sun-dried tomatoes for the grape tomatoes.

Whisk the hummus with the lemon juice, 2 tbsp (30 mL) of the olive oil and pepper. Reserve. Separate the pitas into thin halves and cut into bite-sized wedges. Combine remaining olive oil, paprika and salt and toss with the pita wedges. Toast in a 350°F (180°C) oven, turning once, until golden and crispy, about 10 minutes. Reserve.

Rub a large salad bowl with the garlic clove. Place the lettuce, onion and tomatoes in the bowl. Just before serving, sprinkle the toasted pita wedges over top, add hummus dressing and gently toss to coat. Serve immediately with lemon wedges on the side.

Hummus
If you can't find a great prepared hummus, try whipping up a batch of your own. In a food processor, combine 1 can (19 oz/540 mL) chickpeas, drained and rinsed, 1/2 cup (125 mL) tahini, 3 cloves garlic, 2 tbsp (30 mL) each lemon juice and extra-virgin olive oil, 1/4 tsp (1 mL) ground cumin and salt and freshly ground pepper to taste. Process until smooth and store in the refrigerator for up to 7 days. Makes 2 cups (500 mL).

Mango Tango Slaw

Serves 6

Island-inspired goodness! With a unique coconut mango dressing and loads of crunch and color, this gorgeous slaw will have picnic guests raving.

2 cups	finely shredded green cabbage	500 mL
1 cup	finely shredded red cabbage	250 mL
1 cup	shredded carrot	250 mL
1/2 cup	crushed pineapple, drained	125 mL
1/2 cup	finely chopped green onion	125 mL
2 tbsp	finely chopped cilantro	30 mL

Dressing:

1/2 cup	light coconut milk	125 mL
1/4 cup	sweet mango chutney	60 mL
2 tbsp	fresh lime juice	30 mL
1/2 tsp	hot pepper sauce	2 mL
1/2 tsp	salt	2 mL
1/4 tsp	freshly ground pepper	1 mL

PER SERVING	
Calories	213
Fat (g)	5
Protein (g)	7
Carbohydrate (g)	42
Fiber (g)	9
Sodium (mg)	289

A very high source of fiber. An excellent source of vitamin A, vitamin C, folate, thiamine, pantothenic acid, calcium and magnesium.

Toss together the green and red cabbages, carrot, pineapple, onion and cilantro in a large bowl. Stir the coconut milk with the chutney, lime juice, hot sauce, salt and pepper in a small bowl. Pour the dressing over the cabbage mixture and toss to coat. Cover and reserve in the refrigerator for at least 1 hour before serving to develop the flavors.

Super Slaws

Slaws are an excellent side-dish option for almost any meal, and they don't have to be limited to cabbage and carrots. Other favorite "shreddables" include parsnips, zucchini, broccoli stems, napa cabbage, jicama, kohlrabi, fennel and daikon (Asian radish). Talk to the produce manager in your supermarket for some tips on how to use some of the more exotic vegetables. Shred vegetables quickly and easily using the grater attachment on your food processor or with a mandolin or box grater. Dressings can be creamy or oil and vinegar–based. Try a new combination today!

Diva Pasta Salad

PER SERVING	
Calories	317
Fat (g)	12
Protein (g)	9
Carbohydrate (g)	49
Fiber (g)	6
Sodium (mg)	263

A very high source of fiber. An excellent source of vitamin A, vitamin E and magnesium.

Serves 6

An updated version of an old-fashioned buffet favorite, this salad is a healthy winner—especially for women. The broccoli and almonds contribute calcium, which is important for strong, healthy bones and the prevention of osteoporosis.

1	bunch broccoli, about 1 lb (500 g)	1
2 cups	dry whole-wheat short pasta such as rotini	500 mL
1/2 cup	diced red onion	125 mL
1/2 cup	raisins or dried cranberries	125 mL
1/2 cup	grated carrot	125 mL
1/2 cup	light mayonnaise	125 mL
2 tbsp	granulated sugar	30 mL
1 tbsp	white wine vinegar	15 mL
1 tbsp	lemon juice	15 mL
1/4 tsp	each salt and freshly ground pepper	1 mL
1/2 cup	slivered almonds, toasted	125 mL

Wash the broccoli and trim off the florets, cutting into bite-sized pieces. Reserve. Peel the broccoli stems and chop into bite-sized pieces. Reserve. Cook the pasta according to package directions. During the last 2 minutes of cooking, stir in the broccoli florets and stems. Drain and rinse under cold water.

Combine the broccoli florets and stems, cooked pasta, red onion, raisins, and carrot in a large bowl. In a small bowl, stir together the mayonnaise, sugar, vinegar, lemon juice, salt and pepper until smooth. Pour the dressing over the broccoli mixture and mix well. Sprinkle with almonds just before serving. Store in an airtight container in the refrigerator for up to 2 days.

TIP: To toast the almonds, spread in one layer in a pie plate or baking sheet. Bake in a preheated 350°F (180°C) oven for 5 to 10 minutes or until golden brown and fragrant. Watch carefully and stir often to ensure even browning.

Benefits of Broccoli

Broccoli is a cruciferous vegetable, one of the brassica family of vegetables known to help prevent certain types of cancer. It is also a source of calcium, although the calcium it delivers is not as easily absorbed as that from other sources. A half-cup (125 mL) of raw broccoli contains over 7 grams of fiber. When cooking with broccoli, don't waste the stalk, since it is also full of nutrients. Peel it and chop it into bite-sized pieces to eat raw or cooked, or shred it into salads, slaws and stir-fries.

Indian Princess Salad

Serves 8

PER SERVING	
Calories	282
Fat (g)	12
Protein (g)	10
Carbohydrate (g)	36
Fiber (g)	7
Sodium (mg)	426

A very high source of fiber. An excellent source of vitamin A and folate.

Sweet and tangy, this salad uses canned lentils, which need only to be rinsed before mixing with the rest of the ingredients. Indian-style curry paste is sold in most grocery stores and has a wonderful rich flavor. Combine leftovers with leaf lettuce for a delicious garden wrap for your lunch the next day.

1 cup	whole-wheat couscous	250 mL
1¼ cups	chicken or vegetable broth	300 mL
1	can (19 oz/540 mL) brown lentils, drained and well rinsed	1
1 cup	grated carrot	250 mL
6	green onions, thinly sliced	6
1	red pepper, diced	1
¼ cup	dried currants	60 mL

Dressing:

1 tbsp	mild curry paste or 1 tsp (5 mL) curry powder	15 mL
¼ tsp	ground cumin	1 mL
1 tbsp	brown sugar or honey	15 mL
2 tbsp	white wine vinegar	30 mL
⅓ cup	vegetable oil	75 mL
½ tsp	each salt and freshly ground pepper	2 mL

Place the couscous in a large heatproof bowl. Bring the broth to the boil in a saucepan or in the microwave and pour over the couscous. Cover the bowl and let stand at room temperature for 5 minutes. Uncover the bowl, gently fluff the couscous with a fork and cool to room temperature. Combine the couscous with the lentils, carrot, green onions, red pepper and currants in a large bowl.

Stir together the curry paste, cumin, sugar and vinegar in a small bowl. Whisk in the vegetable oil until combined. Season with salt and pepper. Toss the couscous and vegetables with the dressing. Let stand for 15 minutes before serving. Keeps in the refrigerator for up to 2 days.

Crazy About Couscous

An instant meal-maker, couscous has become common on grocery-store shelves. Although many people consider it a grain, it is actually a pasta made from semolina. Prepared in almost an instant, couscous is delicious in salads and pilafs, as a base for spicy stews or in a wrap sandwich. Change the flavor by using different broths or fruit juice as the cooking liquid. Simply immerse 1 part couscous in 1¼ parts boiling liquid, cover and let stand for 5 minutes before fluffing with a fork. Choose the whole-wheat version over the refined version for higher fiber content—you won't notice a taste difference.

Auckland Chicken Salad

PER SERVING	
Calories	274
Fat (g)	14
Protein (g)	22
Carbohydrate (g)	16
Fiber (g)	4
Sodium (mg)	124

A high source of fiber. An excellent source of vitamin C.

Serves 6

A unique and colorful salad, this can work as a main course or a side dish. It's a perfect way to use up leftover chicken.

3 cups	green beans, about 12 oz (350 g)	750 mL
2	cooked boneless, skinless chicken breasts (about 1 lb/500 g)	2
1	red pepper	1
4	ripe golden or green kiwis	4
1 tbsp	frozen raspberry concentrate, thawed	15 mL
1 tbsp	red wine vinegar	15 mL
2 tsp	whole-grain mustard	10 mL
1/4 tsp	each salt and freshly ground pepper	1 mL
Dash	Worcestershire sauce (optional)	Dash
1/3 cup	olive oil	75 mL
2 tbsp	chopped pecans (optional) toasted (see Tips, pages 40 and 98)	30 mL

Trim the stem ends from the green beans and blanch in a large pot of boiling, salted water for 4 minutes. Drain and run under cold water to stop the cooking process; drain again. Cut the chicken and the red pepper into thin strips. Peel the kiwis and cut into wedges.

Whisk together the raspberry concentrate, vinegar, mustard, salt, pepper and Worcestershire sauce in a small bowl. Whisking constantly, drizzle in the olive oil slowly until the dressing is well combined.

In a large bowl, gently toss the beans, chicken, red pepper and kiwis with the dressing until coated. Sprinkle with toasted pecans, if using, just before serving.

TIP: Add summertime flavor to this salad by brushing two raw chicken breasts with a little of the dressing and grilling over medium-high heat for about 15 minutes, turning once, until cooked through.

Kiwis

Grown in New Zealand and California, kiwis are a source of fiber and an excellent source of vitamin C. Store ripe kiwis in the refrigerator for up to 3 weeks. They can be halved and scooped out like a melon to eat out of your hand or peeled and sliced. Try the new golden kiwis as well as the more common green variety.

Southwestern Supper Salad

Serves 4

Adults and kids alike will enjoy this Tex-Mex-inspired salad. Serve with tortilla chips to crumble over the top or to scoop up the delicious layers. The dressing is wonderfully spicy, but for those with milder tastes, leave out the chipotle pepper or substitute your favorite purchased dressing for a time-saving shortcut.

3/4 cup	buttermilk	175 mL
1/2 cup	light mayonnaise	125 mL
2 tbsp	chopped fresh parsley	30 mL
1	clove garlic, minced	1
1 tbsp	dried onion flakes	15 mL
1 tsp	freshly ground black pepper	5 mL
1/2 tsp	salt	2 mL
1	canned chipotle pepper, seeds discarded, chopped, or 2 tsp/10 mL chipotle pepper sauce	1
1 lb	boneless, skinless chicken breasts	500 g
4 cups	shredded romaine lettuce	1 L
1 cup	canned black or kidney beans, drained and rinsed	250 mL
1 cup	cooked or thawed frozen corn kernels	250 mL
4	green onions, sliced	4
1	tomato, diced	1
2/3 cup	shredded cheddar cheese	150 mL
	Tortilla chips (optional)	

PER SERVING	
Calories	581
Fat (g)	26
Protein (g)	52
Carbohydrate (g)	36
Fiber (g)	7
Sodium (mg)	1162

A very high source of fiber. An excellent source of vitamin A, vitamin D, folate, riboflavin, calcium, magnesium and zinc.

Combine the buttermilk, mayonnaise, parsley, garlic, onion flakes, pepper, salt and chipotle pepper in a blender or food processor. Purée until smooth. Place the chicken breasts in a shallow dish and pour half the marinade over them (reserve the remainder to use as dressing), turn to coat and let stand for 10 minutes at room temperature.

Preheat a grill to medium-high or a broiler to high. Grill or broil the chicken breasts until cooked through, about 15 minutes, turning as needed and brushing with the marinade. Let stand for 5 minutes, then slice thinly at an angle; reserve.

Meanwhile, divide the lettuce between 4 serving plates (or arrange on a large platter) and layer on top the beans, corn, onion, tomato, cheese and sliced chicken. Drizzle with extra dressing and serve with crumbled tortilla chips if desired.

Salad for Supper

In the summer months, when heat and humidity are high, a light salad supper fills the bill. Adding grilled poultry, meat, seafood and legumes contributes to the protein count. Simply marinate the meat in a dressing, then grill and set atop fresh greens and vegetables. Serve with a little extra dressing on the side.

Spoon It Up

Nothing is more comforting than a hearty soup and a loaf of crusty whole-grain bread, especially in the cold winter months. Most soups can be made ahead or even doubled; the extra batch can go into the freezer for a quick winter warm-up.

Heart-Healthy Minestrone

PER SERVING

Calories	313
Fat (g)	5
Protein (g)	18
Carbohydrate (g)	53
Fiber (g)	11
Sodium (mg)	1314

A very high source of fiber.
An excellent source of vitamin A, vitamin D, vitamin C,
folate, niacin, thiamine, iron,
magnesium and zinc.

Serves 6

This big batch of soup is perfect for a winter supper (served with the garlic and herb spelt biscuits on page 109). If making the soup to freeze, leave the pasta out and add it when reheating.

1 tbsp	vegetable oil	15 mL
1	onion, quartered and thinly sliced	1
1 tsp	dried oregano	5 mL
1 tsp	dried basil	5 mL
1 tsp	each salt and freshly ground pepper	5 mL
1/2 tsp	dried thyme	2 mL
1	green pepper, chopped	1
1	zucchini, thinly sliced	1
1	carrot, thinly sliced	1
2 cups	sliced mushrooms	500 mL
1	can (28 oz/796 mL) diced tomatoes	1
1 cup	corn kernels, cooked or thawed	250 mL
1	can (19 oz/540 mL) kidney beans, drained and rinsed	1
5 cups	low-sodium chicken or vegetable broth	1.25 L
1 cup	short whole-wheat pasta such as small shells	250 mL
1 tsp	balsamic vinegar	5 mL
	Grated Parmesan cheese (optional)	

Heat the oil in a large Dutch oven or stockpot. Add onion, oregano, basil, salt, pepper and thyme and cook for 3 minutes or until softened and fragrant. Add green pepper, zucchini, carrot, mushrooms, tomatoes, corn, beans and chicken broth. Bring to the boil. Add the pasta and reduce heat to medium. Simmer, partially covered, for 12 minutes or until the noodles are cooked. Stir in the vinegar just before serving. Serve with Parmesan cheese at the table if desired.

Photo: Pumpernickel
Muffaletta (page 102)

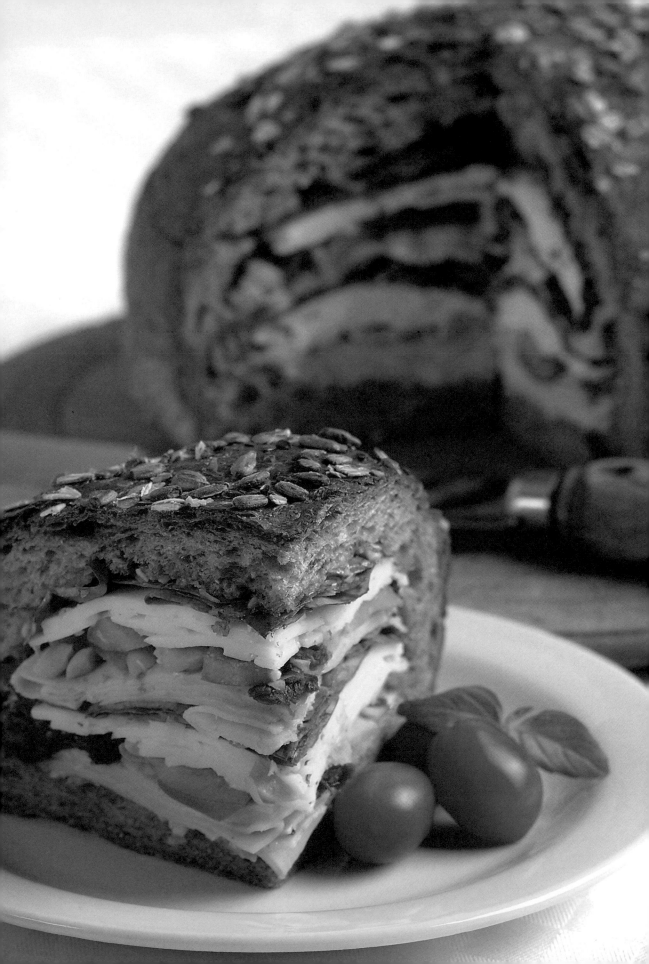

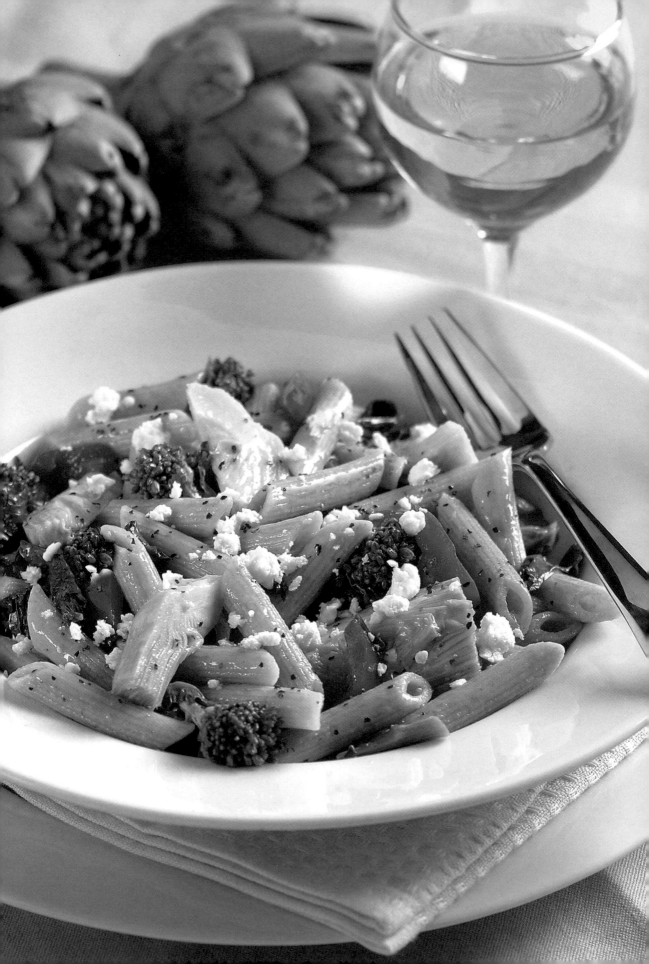

Roasted Parsnip and Pear Soup

Serves 8

A sweetly spiced soup that is the perfect starter for a holiday meal or an elegant dinner party.

1¹/₂ lb	parsnips	750 g
2	pears	2
2 tbsp	vegetable oil, divided	30 mL
2 tsp	mild Indian-style curry paste or powder	10 mL
¹/₂ tsp	each salt and freshly ground pepper	2 mL
1	onion, chopped	1
6 cups	chicken broth (approx.)	1.5 L
1 cup	apple juice	250 mL
1	bay leaf	1
1 tsp	cider vinegar	5 mL
¹/₂ cup	sour cream or yogurt	125 mL
	Chopped fresh chives	

PER SERVING	
Calories	182
Fat (g)	9
Protein (g)	6
Carbohydrate (g)	22
Fiber (g)	4
Sodium (mg)	742

A high source of fiber. An excellent source of folate.

Preheat oven to 375°F (190°C). Scrub and peel the parsnips. Chop into 2-inch (5 cm) chunks. Peel and quarter the pears. Combine 1 tbsp (15 mL) vegetable oil with the curry paste. Toss the parsnips and pears with the curry mixture and sprinkle with salt and pepper. Transfer to a rimmed baking sheet and roast for 45 minutes.

Heat the remaining oil in a large Dutch oven set over medium heat. Add the onion, and cook until beginning to soften, about 4 minutes. Add the roasted parsnips and pears, chicken broth, apple juice and bay leaf. Bring the soup to the boil and simmer for 10 to 15 minutes.

Purée the soup in batches in a blender or food processor until smooth. Return to pot, stir in the vinegar and season with salt and pepper to taste. If the soup is too thick for your taste, add a little extra chicken broth and simmer for a few minutes. Just before serving, whisk in the sour cream or yogurt until well blended. Sprinkle with chives and serve.

TIP: For a fancier presentation, drizzle a little extra sour cream or yogurt over the top of the soup and garnish with fresh chives.

Photo: Italian Flag Pasta (page 70)

Roasted Goodness

Roasting vegetables allows the exterior sugars of the vegetables to caramelize, adding a flavor dimension that is lacking in boiled vegetables. Roasting also maintains more nutrients (they aren't thrown out with the cooking water). Try roasting hearty winter vegetables such as squash, rutabaga, carrots and potatoes. Toss them with a little oil and flavorful herbs, then eat as is, turn into a mash or purée with some broth for a thick and hearty soup. Puréeing root vegetables adds bulk to soups and eliminates the need for other thickeners.

Ginger Chicken Soup with Soba Noodles

Serves 4

Trade in boring old chicken noodle soup for this updated Asian-inspired version. Buckwheat soba noodles add fiber and gourmet appeal. The broth is infused with fresh ginger, which has tummy-soothing properties that will make this substantial noodle bowl your new comfort soup.

1	bunch green onions, about 6	1
1	bone-in, skinless chicken breast (about ¹/₂ lb/250 g)	1
1	2-inch (5 cm) piece raw ginger, sliced	1
2	cans (each 10 oz/284 mL) low-sodium chicken broth	2
4 cups	water	1 L
4 oz	soba (buckwheat) noodles or whole-wheat spaghettini	125 g
1	red pepper, cut into strips	1
1	carrot, cut into thin sticks	1
1	stalk celery, cut thinly on the diagonal	1
1 tbsp	soy sauce	15 mL
¹/₂ tsp	hot pepper sauce (optional)	2 mL
¹/₄ tsp	sesame oil	1 mL
1 tsp	toasted sesame seeds (optional)	5 mL

PER SERVING	
Calories	218
Fat (g)	4
Protein (g)	25
Carbohydrate (g)	23
Fiber (g)	4
Sodium (mg)	1076

A high source of fiber. An excellent source of vitamin A, vitamin C and folate.

Recipe Makeover: Classic chicken noodle soup gets a fiber boost with nutty buckwheat noodles and colorful vegetables.

Coarsely chop 4 of the green onions; reserve the remainder for the garnish. Combine the chopped onions with the chicken, ginger, broth and water in a large pot. Bring to the boil over medium-high heat and simmer for 15 minutes, partially covered. Strain and reserve the broth and chicken but discard the onions and ginger. Cut the chicken from the bone and slice thinly, set in a bowl and cover to keep warm.

Return the broth to the pot and bring to the boil. Add the noodles and cook for 2 minutes. Stir in the red pepper strips, carrot and celery and cook for 3 minutes more. Stir in the soy sauce, hot pepper sauce, if using, and sesame oil.

Use a slotted spoon to transfer equal portions of noodles and vegetables into 4 serving bowls. Top with sliced chicken and pour equal amounts of the hot broth into each bowl. Thinly slice the remaining green onions and sprinkle over soup. Sprinkle with toasted sesame seeds, if using. Serve with a fork for twirling up the noodles and a spoon for slurping up the broth.

Buckwheat, or soba, noodles, an essential ingredient in Japanese cooking, are becoming more common in North America. This is good news, because not only do quick-cooking soba noodles taste fabulous but they are also high in protein and fiber; some brands are gluten-free for those who have celiac disease or gluten intolerance.

Fiber Boost: Everyday Cooking for a Long, Healthy Life

Wild Woods Soup

Serves 6

This robust soup made with wild mushrooms, wild rice and golden squash will reinvent the way you look at mushroom soup. The intensity of the mushroom flavor will depend on the types of mushrooms used.

1 lb	mixed wild mushrooms (such as cremini, portobello, shiitake and oyster)	500 g
1 tbsp	olive oil	15 mL
1	large sweet onion, thinly sliced	1
2	cloves garlic, minced	2
1 tsp	ground cumin	5 mL
1 tsp	Worcestershire sauce	5 mL
1 cup	cooked wild rice	250 mL
2 cups	shredded butternut squash (about 12 oz/350 g)	500 mL
4 cups	beef broth	1 L
1/2 cup	dry white wine	125 mL

PER SERVING	
Calories	196
Fat (g)	3
Protein (g)	9
Carbohydrate (g)	33
Fiber (g)	4
Sodium (mg)	546

A high source of fiber. An excellent source of vitamin A, vitamin D, folate, niacin and zinc.

Brush away any dirt clinging to the mushrooms and slice thinly. (Discard the stems of the shiitakes, if using, because they are tough.) Heat the olive oil in a Dutch oven or large saucepan set over medium heat. Add the onion and garlic and cook for 3 minutes or until softened.

Add the mushrooms and cumin to the pot and cook, stirring often, for 8 minutes or until browned. Stir in the Worcestershire sauce, wild rice, squash, broth and wine. Bring to the boil and simmer for 10 minutes or until the squash is tender.

Bistro White Bean Soup

PER SERVING

Calories	308
Fat (g)	9
Protein (g)	21
Carbohydrate (g)	38
Fiber (g)	10
Sodium (mg)	1391

A very high source of fiber.
An excellent source of vitamin A, folate, thiamine, iron,
magnesium and zinc.

Serves 4

A rustic winter soup accented with smoky bacon and topped with delicious cheesey croutons. Serve this bistro-style soup on a snowy day, and you'll be a big hit.

1 tbsp	olive oil	15 mL
4 oz	bacon, chopped	125 g
1	large onion, chopped	1
2	carrots, diced	2
2	cloves garlic, minced	2
1 tsp	dried thyme	5 mL
1/2 tsp	each salt and freshly ground pepper	2 mL
1	bay leaf	1
2	cans (each 19 oz/540 mL) white kidney beans, drained and rinsed	2
4 cups	chicken broth	1 L
4 cups	baby spinach	1 L

Parmesan-Pepper Croutons:

2	thick slices whole-grain bread	2
1 tbsp	olive oil	15 mL
2 tbsp	finely grated Parmesan cheese	30 mL
1 tsp	freshly ground pepper	5 mL

Heat the olive oil in a large Dutch oven or saucepan set over medium heat. Add the bacon and cook until browned and slightly crisp. Stir in the onion, carrots, garlic, thyme, salt, pepper and bay leaf. Cook, stirring often, for 10 minutes or until tender and golden. Add the beans and chicken broth and bring the soup to the boil. Reduce the heat and simmer for 20 minutes.

Remove the bay leaf. Use a potato masher or the back of a spoon to crush some of the beans to thicken the soup. Stir in the spinach and cook just until wilted. Ladle the soup into bowls and serve with Parmesan-pepper croutons.

Parmesan-Pepper Croutons:
Preheat the oven to 350°F (180°C). Cut the bread into 1-inch (2.5 cm) cubes and, in a large bowl, toss with the olive oil, Parmesan cheese and pepper. Spread out on a foil-lined baking sheet and bake for 10 minutes or until golden and toasted.

Legumes

Although canned legumes are easy to work with, some people prefer to use dried. They are very shelf-stable and, when cooked, have a lower sodium content than their canned counterparts.

Dried legumes need to be soaked before cooking; there are two methods:
- Long Soak: Cover dried beans with 3 to 4 times their volume of water, allow to stand 4 to 8 hours or overnight. Drain and rinse well.
- Quick Soak: Cover dried beans with 3 to 4 times their volume of water, bring to a boil and simmer for 2 minutes. Remove from heat and let stand 1 hour. Drain and rinse well.

To cook, cover the beans with $2^1/_2$ times their volume of fresh water and bring to the boil. Reduce the heat and simmer until tender. Cooking times will vary depending on the bean. One cup (250 mL) dried beans generally yields $2^1/_2$ cups (625 mL) cooked. See the chart below for the cooking times for some common beans.

Legume	Approx. Cooking Time
Adzuki or small red beans	40 to 50 minutes
Black beans	$1^3/_4$ hours
Black-eyed peas	50 to 60 minutes
Great northern beans	60 minutes
Green or brown lentils	30 minutes
Lima beans	20 minutes
Navy (pea) beans	50 minutes
Pinto beans	45 minutes
Red kidney beans	60 minutes
Red lentils	10 minutes
Soy beans	$3^1/_2$ to 4 hours
Split yellow or green peas	75 minutes
White kidney beans	40 minutes

Won't Miss the Meat-Less Chili

PER SERVING

Calories	295
Fat (g)	4
Protein (g)	21
Carbohydrate (g)	51
Fiber (g)	8
Sodium (mg)	1586

A very high source of fiber. An excellent source of vitamin A, vitamin B$_6$, vitamin C, vitamin D, vitamin E, folate, thiamine, iron and magnesium.

Recipe Makeover:

Traditional chili gets an even greater fiber boost from soy meat alternative, which is lower in fat than beef and is also suitable for vegetarians.

Serves 6

This recipe makes a big batch of home-style chili that is great to take for lunches or to freeze for a busy weeknight supper. Serve with whole-wheat toast or over rice for a hearty meat-free supper.

1 tbsp	vegetable oil	15 mL
1	medium onion, chopped	1
1	clove garlic, minced	1
1	green pepper, diced	1
2 cups	sliced mushrooms (optional)	500 mL
1 tbsp	chili powder	15 mL
2 tsp	dried oregano	10 mL
1 tsp	ground cumin	5 mL
1	can (28 oz/796 mL) diced tomatoes	1
2$^1/_2$ cups	plain tomato sauce	625 mL
1	can (10 oz/284 mL) beans in tomato sauce	1
1	can (14 oz/398 mL) kidney beans	1
1 cup	corn kernels	250 mL
1	package (12 oz/350 g) seasoned soy meat alternative (such as Veggie Ground Round)	1
	Sour cream (optional)	
	Chopped fresh cilantro (optional)	

Heat the oil in a Dutch oven set over medium-high heat. Add the onion and cook for 2 minutes or until softened. Add the garlic, green pepper and mushrooms and cook for 5 minutes or until vegetables are tender. Add the spices and cook for 1 minute or until fragrant.

Stir in the tomatoes, tomato sauce, beans and corn. Bring to the boil, reduce the heat to medium-low and simmer for 10 minutes. Crumble the meat alternative into the chili and cook until just heated through, about 5 minutes. Serve with sour cream and sprinkle with chopped cilantro if desired.

Soy Delicious

For variety, seasoned soy meat alternatives make an excellent fiber-rich substitute for ground meat in hearty dishes such as chili. They are often fat-free, preservative-free, protein-rich and fortified with vitamins and minerals. Most soy alternatives do not need to be cooked like ground meats, just heated through. The seasoned soy products may contain more salt, so if you want to control your salt intake, you can make your own version by hydrating dry textured vegetable protein (TVP) with your own seasoned broth. (See page 28 for more information on TVP.)

Sensational Sides

Jazz up your plate with these spectacular and tasty side dishes.

These recipes are perfect for any night of the week:

Smashed Potatoes, Pass Them On

Perfect Pilaf

Flamin' Red Beans

Chili-Lime Corn Skillet

Spiced Sweet Potato Fries

If you're looking for a make-ahead dish for holidays or potlucks, these recipes fill the bill:

Rutabaga, Parsnip and Apple Crumble

Cauliflower Gratin

Sugar-Bush Brussels Sprouts

Roasted Fennel and Three Peppers

Smashed Potatoes, Pass Them On

Recipe Makeover:
Roasting the skins until crispy adds delicious texture as well as a fiber boost to your (s)mashed potatoes.

Serves 4

Traditional mashed potatoes call for peeling potatoes and then boiling them until they are tender. Often the result is a soggy, flavorless mound that screams for butter to help. Instead of peeling the extra fiber away, leave the peel on, infuse the potatoes with flavored oil and roast until crispy before smashing into creamy goodness. Start with 1½ lb (750 g) of new red- or white-skinned potatoes. Scrub well to remove any dirt, trim away blemishes and dry thoroughly. Cut large potatoes in half.

Preheat oven to 375°F (190°C). Following the chart below, toss the potatoes in a large bowl with "Flavoring Ingredients" and add any "Extras" listed. Transfer to an ungreased roasting pan and roast, uncovered and stirring often, for 40 minutes, or until crispy on the outside and tender on the inside. (Extra ingredients such as garlic and fruit may become quite soft and browned; this will add delicious flavour.) Scrape the contents of the roasting pan into a bowl. Smash the roasted potatoes with the "Smashing Liquids" and season to taste with salt and pepper. Serve immediately.

	Flavoring Ingredients	Extras	Smashing Liquids
1. Sea Salt and Pepper	2 tbsp (30 mL) olive oil 2 tsp (10 mL) coarse sea salt 2 tsp (10 ml) freshly ground pepper		⅔ cup (150 mL) buttermilk
2. Roasted Garlic and Apple	2 tbsp (30 mL) olive oil ½ tsp (2 mL) dried thyme	2 apples, peeled and halved 8 whole garlic cloves, peeled and roasted	½ cup (125 mL) fat-free sour cream
3. Chili-Ranch	2 tbsp (30 mL) canola oil 2 tsp (10 mL) chili powder ½ tsp (2 mL) dried oregano		⅔ cup (150 mL) light ranch dressing 2 tbsp (30 mL) freshly grated Parmesan cheese
4. Bistro Blue Cheese	2 tbsp (30 mL) olive oil 1 tsp (5 mL) dried rosemary	8 whole garlic cloves, peeled and finely chopped	½ cup (125 mL) light sour cream ¼ cup (60 mL) crumbled blue cheese

Fiber Boost: Leave the Skins On!

Whenever possible, scrub root vegetables such as carrots, potatoes and sweet potatoes to remove surface dirt and blemishes, but leave the skins on. Because it has the job of holding the vegetable together, the skin often contains more fiber than the softer interior. Roasting vegetables is the perfect choice for skins-on cooking, making the exterior nice and crispy and the inside tender.

Perfect Pilaf

Serves 4

The pilaf method of cooking is a versatile one, allowing for a range of grains and flavoring ingredients. Use the table opposite for ideas to create the perfect accompaniment to your next meal.

1 tbsp	vegetable oil	15 mL
1 tbsp	butter	15 mL
1/2 cup	chopped onion	125 mL
1	stalk celery, minced	1
1/2 cup	grated carrot	125 mL
1 tsp	dried thyme	5 mL
1 cup	long-grain brown rice, brown and wild rice mix, bulgur, quinoa, barley* or couscous*	250 mL
2 cups	chicken or vegetable broth	500 mL

Heat the oil and butter in a large nonstick skillet set over medium heat. Add the onion, celery, carrot and thyme and cook until tender and fragrant, about 5 minutes. Add the rice (or other grain) and stir until coated with the oil and seasonings. Stir in the chicken broth and bring to the boil. Reduce the heat to low, cover and cook until all the fluid is absorbed and the grains are tender to the bite. Fluff with a fork and serve.

* If using barley, increase the broth to 3 cups (750 mL); if using couscous, decrease the broth to 1¼ cups (300 mL).

Variations:

Apple Orchard Pilaf: Substitute 1 cup (250 mL) diced fresh or dried apple for the celery and carrot. Replace 1 cup (250 mL) of the broth with apple juice.

Wild Mushroom Pilaf: Substitute 2 cups (500 mL) chopped wild mushrooms for the celery and carrot. Stir 1 tbsp (15 mL) balsamic vinegar into the broth.

Orange Cranberry Pilaf: Substitute 1 cup (250 mL) dried cranberries for the celery and carrot. Replace 1 cup (250 mL) of the broth with orange juice.

Use this table when experimenting with different grains:

Grain	Volume of Liquid (per 1 cup/250 mL grain)	Cooking Time
Brown and wild rice blend	2 cups (500 mL)	35 minutes
Buckwheat, or kasha*	2 cups (500 mL)	15 minutes
Bulgur	2 cups (500 mL)	20 minutes
Couscous	1$\frac{1}{4}$ cups (300 mL)	5 minutes
Long-grain brown rice	2 cups (500 mL)	35 minutes
Old-fashioned oats*	$\frac{3}{4}$ cup (175 mL)	3 minutes
Pearl barley	3 cups (750 mL)	40 minutes
Pot barley	3$\frac{1}{2}$ cups (875 mL)	45 minutes
Quinoa	2 cups (500 mL)	15 minutes
Wheat or spelt berries (soaked overnight)	4 cups (1 L)	60 minutes

* To keep grains firm and separate, toss with 1 beaten egg and allow to toast well in the pan before adding the liquid.

Flamin' Red Beans

PER SERVING	
Calories	120
Fat (g)	3
Protein (g)	6
Carbohydrate (g)	20
Fiber (g)	5
Sodium (mg)	143

A very high source of fiber. An excellent source of vitamin C and folate.

Serves 6

A quick and fiery side dish for times when you want something different. The crimson color of the kidney beans looks great on the plate!

1 tbsp	vegetable oil	15 mL
1/2 cup	chopped yellow pepper	125 mL
1/2 cup	chopped red onion	125 mL
1 tsp	Asian chili paste such as sambal olek (or to taste)	5 mL
1 tbsp	brown sugar	15 mL
1 tbsp	lime juice	15 mL
1	can (14 oz/398 mL) kidney beans, drained and rinsed	1

Heat the oil in a nonstick skillet set over medium-high heat. Add the pepper and onion and stir-fry for 2 to 3 minutes or until tender. In a separate bowl, stir together chili paste, sugar and lime juice. Add to the pan and cook, stirring, for 1 minute or until fragrant.

Add the beans and cook for about 2 minutes more or until heated through and coated with sauce. Serve warm or at room temperature.

TIP: If you can't find Asian Chili paste, add your favorite hot pepper sauce to taste.

Love Those Legumes

Eating legumes as a side dish can add flavor as well as fiber to any meal. Canned legumes are easy to prepare and can be enhanced with spices, herbs and vinaigrettes to add extra flair. To reduce salt and the unpleasant side effects that can accompany canned beans, drain and rinse them well before adding to your recipes.

Chili-Lime Corn Skillet

Serves 6

Jazz up boring frozen corn kernels in this zippy side dish. Simply pull them out of the freezer and pop them into the skillet. Adding red cabbage makes for a surprising combination that is both flavorful and colorful.

1 tbsp	vegetable oil	15 mL
2 cups	frozen corn kernels	500 mL
1 cup	very finely shredded red cabbage	250 mL
1/2 cup	green onions, sliced	125 mL
1 tbsp	chili powder	15 mL
1 tsp	finely grated lime peel	5 mL
1 tbsp	fresh lime juice	15 mL
1/2 tsp	each salt and freshly ground pepper	2 mL

PER SERVING	
Calories	168
Fat (g)	4
Protein (g)	6
Carbohydrate (g)	33
Fiber (g)	7
Sodium (mg)	240

A very high source of fiber. An excellent source of vitamin C, folate and magnesium.

Heat the oil in a large skillet set over medium-high heat. Add the corn and cabbage and cook, stirring often, until the corn is golden and the cabbage is wilted, about 3 minutes. Stir in the green onions, chili powder, lime peel, juice, salt and pepper. Cook, stirring, for 1 minute or until the mixture is well coated and heated through.

Dynamic Duos

Add variety to your plate with these vegetable (and legume) combos:

- Whole cooked green or yellow beans tossed with chopped fresh tomato and a vinaigrette made of whole-grain mustard, red wine vinegar and vegetable oil
- Mushrooms sautéed with spinach and garlic butter
- Cauliflower (blanched) and cooked green peas tossed with curry paste and butter
- Zucchini and red pepper sautéed with lemon and butter
- Thinly sliced raw or sautéed carrot and celery tossed with French-style dressing

Spiced Sweet Potato Fries

PER SERVING	
Calories	314
Fat (g)	7
Protein (g)	4
Carbohydrate (g)	60
Fiber (g)	7
Sodium (mg)	601

A very high source of fiber. An excellent source of vitamin A, vitamin C, vitamin B$_6$ and folate.

Recipe Makeover: Oven-baked sweet potatoes with the skins left on provide a much greater fiber boost (as well as antioxidants) than traditional starchy, fat-laden fries.

Serves 4

When I was at university, the smell of pineapple-glazed sweet potato fries would waft across the commons, teasing me on my way to class. These are much classier than traditional fries, and there's no need to pass the ketchup!

$^1/_2$ cup	unsweetened pineapple juice	125 mL
1 tsp	each ground ginger and ground cinnamon	5 mL
$^1/_4$ tsp	paprika	1 mL
1 tsp	salt	5 mL
$^1/_2$ tsp	freshly ground pepper	2 mL
4	medium sweet potatoes (about 2 lb/1 kg)	4
2 tbsp	vegetable oil	30 mL

Heat the pineapple juice in a small saucepan set over medium-high heat. Bring to the boil, then simmer over medium heat until syrupy (about one-quarter its original volume). Stir in the ginger, cinnamon, paprika, salt and pepper and cool slightly.

Preheat the oven to 425°F (220°C). Scrub the sweet potatoes and dry completely but do not peel. Cut into long, thin wedges, spread out on paper towels and blot dry. Heat the oil on a baking sheet in the oven for 5 to 6 minutes or until very hot and smoking. Carefully spread the sweet potatoes out in a single layer in the heated pan and bake until crispy on the outside and tender on the inside, about 30 minutes, stirring as needed. Just before serving, drizzle with the pineapple glaze.

TIP: For the crispiest oven fries, be sure that the pan is smoking when you put the potatoes in it and that the vegetables are well-spaced in a single layer. Use an extra baking sheet if necessary.

Sweet Potatoes

Sweet potatoes are high in fiber and vitamins A and C. They are sometimes called yams, although real yams are rarely sold in Canadian stores and are much less sweet than the vibrant colored sweet potatoes we are accustomed to. Choose medium, unblemished sweet potatoes and store in a cool dark dry place. You can substitute sweet potatoes for regular potatoes in many recipes.

Rutabaga, Parsnip and Apple Crumble

Serves 8

Even people who typically don't like rutabaga will enjoy this tasty version with apple chunks and a sweet crumb topping. It is also a wonderful make-ahead holiday side dish.

4 cups	peeled and cubed rutabaga (about 1½ lb/750 g)	1 L
3 cups	peeled and cubed parsnips (about 1 lb/500 g)	750 mL
½ cup	unsweetened applesauce	125 mL
1 tsp	each salt and freshly ground pepper	5 mL
4	apples, peeled and chopped	4
1 tsp	ground cinnamon	5 mL
1 tsp	ground ginger	5 mL

Topping:

⅓ cup	whole-wheat flour	75 mL
⅓ cup	old-fashioned rolled oats	75 mL
2 tbsp	brown sugar	30 mL
1 tsp	ground cinnamon	5 mL
3 tbsp	cold butter, cubed	45 mL

PER SERVING	
Calories	250
Fat (g)	6
Protein (g)	4
Carbohydrate (g)	49
Fiber (g)	6
Sodium (mg)	364

A very high source of fiber. An excellent source of vitamin C, folate and magnesium.

Preheat the oven to 350°F (180°C). Combine the rutabaga and parsnips in a large pot. Cover with salted water and bring to the boil over medium-high heat. Cover the pot and reduce the heat to medium. Simmer for 20 minutes or until just fork-tender. Drain, reserving ½ cup (125 mL) of the liquid. Mash the vegetables with a potato masher or a hand mixer until smooth. Add the applesauce, salt and pepper and some of the reserved liquid if dry. Toss the apples with cinnamon and ginger. Spread half the rutabaga mixture in a 9- × 13-inch (3L) casserole and top with half the apples. Repeat the layers.

Topping:
Combine flour, oats, brown sugar and cinnamon. With a fork or pastry blender, cut in butter until crumbly. Sprinkle the crumb mixture evenly over the top of the casserole. (Can be prepared up to this point and reserved for 1 day in the refrigerator or for 1 month in the freezer. Thaw before baking and add 5 minutes to the cooking time.) Bake for 30 minutes or until heated through and topping is crisp and brown.

Cauliflower Gratin

PER SERVING	
Calories	191
Fat (g)	13
Protein (g)	9
Carbohydrate (g)	13
Fiber (g)	5
Sodium (mg)	422

A high source of fiber. An excellent source of vitamin C, vitamin D and folate.

Serves 6

Beautiful crumb-topped wedges of cauliflower make an impressive centerpiece at any festive table. I serve them on a platter surrounded by blanched green beans.

1	large head cauliflower (about 2 lb/1 kg)	1
1/4 cup	Dijon mustard	60 mL
1/4 cup	light mayonnaise	60 mL
1/4 cup	finely chopped red pepper	60 mL
2 tbsp	chopped sun-dried tomatoes	30 mL
1/2 cup	shredded sharp cheddar cheese	125 mL
2/3 cup	coarsely crushed bran flake-style cereal	150 mL
2 tbsp	chopped fresh parsley	30 mL
2 tbsp	grated Parmesan cheese	30 mL
1 tsp	finely grated lemon peel	5 mL
1 tbsp	fresh lemon juice	15 mL
1 tbsp	melted butter	15 mL

Wash the cauliflower and remove any blemished spots with a paring knife. Trim off the leaves but leave the stem end intact. Add about 2 inches (5 cm) of water to a pot large enough to hold the cauliflower upright. Bring water to a boil over medium-high heat. Set the cauliflower in the pot, stem side down, and steam for about 8 minutes, covered. Carefully remove the head onto a rimmed baking sheet. Cool, then cut into large wedges; include some of the stem in each wedge to keep the shape. Set the wedges in a 9-inch (23 cm) pie plate, stems facing in.

Preheat the oven to 375°F (190°C). Stir the mustard, mayonnaise, red pepper and sun-dried tomatoes together. Blend in the cheddar. Smear the mixture over the top of the cauliflower wedges. Blend the bran cereal with the parsley, Parmesan, lemon peel, juice and melted butter until crumbly. Sprinkle evenly over the top of the wedges. Bake for 15 minutes or until the topping is golden and bubbly. Serve immediately.

Tip-Toppers

Adding a fiber-rich crumb topping gives crunch and pizzazz to any casserole, vegetable dish or fruit bake. Toss the following with a little melted butter or vegetable oil to make the topping crisp and golden:
- Crushed bran, wheat or granola cereals
- Whole-wheat, rye, pumpernickel or other fiber-rich breadcrumbs
- Chopped nuts such as almonds, pecans and walnuts
- Crushed corn chips

Sugar-Bush Brussels Sprouts

Serves 6

Vibrant green Brussels sprouts are one of the brassicas, a group of vegetables known to have cancer-fighting properties. Instead of using cheese sauce, try this sweet and tangy strategy for preparing the vegetable that kids love to hate.

1 1/2 lb	Brussels sprouts	750 g
1/4 tsp	salt	1 mL
2 tbsp	butter	30 mL
1/4 cup	maple syrup	60 mL
1/4 cup	whole-grain Dijon mustard	60 mL
1 tbsp	fresh lemon juice	15 mL
1/2 tsp	freshly ground pepper	2 mL

PER SERVING	
Calories	120
Fat (g)	5
Protein (g)	3
Carbohydrate (g)	20
Fiber (g)	4
Sodium (mg)	275

A very high source of fiber. An excellent source of calcium, vitamin D and folate.

Bring a large pot of salted water to the boil. Trim the tips off the ends of the sprouts, and remove any blemished leaves. Cut the sprouts in half. Add to the boiling water and blanch for 6 minutes. Drain, then cool quickly under cold running water to stop the cooking process. Drain again and reserve.

Melt the butter in a large skillet set over medium-high heat. Add the maple syrup, mustard and lemon juice, and stir until bubbly and hot, about 1 minute. Add the sprouts and cook, stirring, for 3 minutes, or until glazed and lightly browned. Sprinkle with ground pepper and serve immediately.

TIP: To prepare Brussels sprouts ahead, blanch and cool the sprouts. Melt the butter in a small saucepan or in the microwave. Combine the butter with the maple syrup, mustard and lemon juice. Toss the Brussels sprouts with the mustard mixture and turn into a shallow greased casserole. Reserve in refrigerator for up to 1 day. Bake in a preheated 350°F (180°C) oven for 20 minutes.

Blanching Vegetables

Ever wonder how restaurants keep their vegetables so crisp and colorful? The trick is to avoid overcooking them. Start by bringing a very large pot of salted water to the boil (the salt helps maintain the color of the vegetables). Blanch the vegetables for 1 to 6 minutes, depending on size and desired doneness. It is also important to keep the water at a rolling boil during the cooking time. Remove the vegetables from the water and immediately plunge them into a large bowl of ice water. This stops the cooking process and locks in the wonderful color and crispness. This technique is ideal for asparagus, green and yellow beans, broccoli and many other vegetable favorites.

Roasted Fennel and Three Peppers

PER SERVING	
Calories	108
Fat (g)	0
Protein (g)	3
Carbohydrate (g)	25
Fiber (g)	6
Sodium (mg)	236

A very high source of fiber. An excellent source of vitamin A, vitamin B_6, vitamin C and folate.

Serves 6

An underused vegetable, fennel has a unique licorice flavor that mellows as it is cooked. The addition of peppers make this side dish a colorful accompaniment to any meal.

1	bulb fennel	1
1/2 cup	chicken broth	125 mL
1/4 tsp	each salt and freshly ground pepper	2 mL
1	each red, yellow and green peppers, sliced	1
1	onion, sliced	1
1/4 cup	melted red-pepper jelly	60 mL
1 tbsp	cider vinegar	15 mL
1 tbsp	chopped fresh thyme	15 mL

Cut the tough stem ends off the fennel bulb and use a vegetable peeler to remove any discolored areas on the surface. Cut the bulb into quarters and slice thinly. Heat the chicken broth in an ovenproof skillet set over medium-high heat. Add the fennel and sprinkle with salt and pepper. Cover, turn the heat to low and simmer for 20 minutes. Drain and reserve.

Preheat the oven to 350°F (180°C). Add the peppers and onion to the fennel. Stir together the jelly, vinegar and thyme and toss with vegetable mixture. Transfer to a 7- × 11-inch (2 L) casserole. (Can be prepared up to this point, covered and reserved in refrigerator for 1 day.) Place in the middle of the preheated oven. Roast, stirring occasionally, for 30 minutes or until vegetables are tender.

Fabulous Fennel

Fennel, or anise, is one of my favorite vegetables. With a celery-like texture and a delicious licorice flavor, it is great raw or cooked in salads, pasta dishes, stews, soups and stir-fries.

Pass Me the Pasta

My own personal weeknight staple and a favorite last-minute-company cupboard grab, pasta seems to please everyone. Start with making a simple switch to whole-wheat pastas, then add even more nutritional benefits with vegetable-rich sauces.

Italian Flag Pasta

PER SERVING

Calories	424
Fat (g)	18
Protein (g)	13
Carbohydrate (g)	56
Fiber (g)	8
Sodium (mg)	234

A very high source of fiber. An excellent source of vitamin A, vitamin C, vitamin E, folate, thiamine and magnesium.

Serves 4

Red, green and white vegetables are the highlight of this simple pantry-based pasta dish. It tastes just as good cold as it does warm, so pack up the leftovers for tomorrow's lunch.

2 cups	whole-wheat penne or rotini	500 mL
3 cups	lightly packed chopped rapini	750 mL
1	jar (6 oz/170 mL) marinated artichoke hearts	1
4	roasted red peppers from a jar	4
2 tbsp	extra-virgin olive oil	30 mL
4	cloves garlic, minced	4
1/4 cup	dry white wine	60 mL
2 tsp	Dijon mustard	10 mL
2 tsp	liquid honey	10 mL
1/4 cup	crumbled feta or grated parmesan cheese (optional)	60 mL
	Salt and freshly ground pepper	

Cook the pasta in a large pot of boiling, salted water according to package directions. During the last 4 minutes of cooking, add the rapini. Drain pasta and rapini and keep warm.

Drain the artichoke hearts, reserving the liquid, and chop into bite-sized pieces. Blot the roasted red peppers dry and chop into bite-sized pieces.

Heat the oil in a large skillet set over medium heat. Add the garlic and cook for 1 minute or until fragrant. Stir in the reserved artichoke liquid, wine, mustard and honey. Bring to the boil and reduce heat. Stir in the artichoke hearts, red peppers, pasta and rapini and cook, stirring, until heated through, about 3 minutes. Sprinkle with feta cheese, if using, and season with salt and pepper to taste.

Rapini

With its unique slightly bitter flavor, rapini, or broccoli rabe, is gaining popularity in North American supermarkets. Resembling a leafy version of broccoli, it can be used in a similar fashion. Like broccoli, it is one of the brassicas, so it contains phytochemicals that help prevent cancer.

Dilly Salmon Pasta Primavera

Serves 4

A healthy pantry and freezer provide this quick pasta dish that is rich not only in fiber but in calcium as well. Be sure to crush the bones from the canned salmon and stir them into the sauce for a real calcium boost.

2 cups	dry whole-wheat penne or rotini	500 mL
1 cup	frozen peas	250 mL
2 cups	frozen California-style mixed vegetables	500 mL
	(broccoli, cauliflower and carrots)	
1	can (7^1/$_2$ oz/213 g) sockeye or pink salmon	1
1 tbsp	butter	15 mL
^{1}/$_4$ cup	finely chopped onion	60 mL
1 cup	milk	250 mL
8 oz	light brick-style cream cheese, cubed	250 g
1^1/$_2$ tsp	dried dillweed	7 mL
1 cup	shredded light Swiss cheese	250 mL

Cook the penne according to the package directions. Add the peas and California mix during the last 4 minutes of cooking time. Drain and keep warm. Remove the skin from the salmon and separate into chunks.

Melt the butter in a large skillet set over medium heat. Stir in the onion and cook until just softened, about 2 minutes. Add milk, cream cheese and dill, stirring until the cream cheese is melted and the mixture is bubbly. Stir in the pasta, vegetables, salmon chunks and Swiss cheese. Toss gently until the cheese is melted and the pasta is well coated with sauce.

Supermarket Shortcuts

Take advantage of convenience foods available in the supermarket to cut down on meal preparations such as cutting and washing. Having frozen vegetable blends on hand to throw into pastas, soups and stews or simply to heat for a quick side dish can ease your dinnertime burden.

PER SERVING	
Calories	737
Fat (g)	36
Protein (g)	50
Carbohydrate (g)	56
Fiber (g)	6
Sodium (mg)	1189

A very high source of fiber. An excellent source of vitamin A, vitamin C, vitamin D, vitamin E, folate, niacin, thiamine, riboflavin, calcium, iron, phosphorus, magnesium and zinc.

Black Bean, Beef and Pepper Toss

PER SERVING	
Calories	513
Fat (g)	13
Protein (g)	44
Carbohydrate (g)	58
Fiber (g)	7
Sodium (mg)	304

A very high source of fiber. An excellent source of vitamin A, vitamin C, vitamin B$_6$, vitamin B$_{12}$, thiamine, riboflavin, iron, phosphorus, zinc and magnesium.

Serves 4

This recipe is adapted from a delicious eggplant recipe by Dana McCauley. I loved the sauce so much I incorporated it into this quick stir-fry supper. Look for the fermented black-bean and garlic sauce in your supermarket's Asian-food section.

1	Asian or small (baby) eggplant	1
1 tbsp	vegetable oil	15 mL
1 tsp	sesame oil	5 mL
1 lb	sirloin steak, thinly sliced	500 g
1	small red onion, sliced	1
1	green pepper, thinly sliced	1
1	yellow pepper, thinly sliced	1
1/3 cup	fermented black-bean and garlic sauce	75 mL
2 tbsp	liquid honey	30 mL
2 tsp	finely grated fresh ginger	10 mL
1 tbsp	fresh lime juice	15 mL
2 tbsp	chopped fresh cilantro	30 mL
1 tbsp	toasted sesame seeds	15 mL
4 cups	cooked brown-rice noodles or whole-wheat spaghetti	1 L
	Lime wedges	

Trim the eggplant and cut into ¾-inch (2 cm) cubes. Heat the vegetable oil and sesame oil in a large skillet or wok set over medium-high heat. Add the beef and stir-fry until browned all over. Remove from the skillet and reserve. Add the eggplant, onion and pepper strips to the pan and stir-fry for 5 minutes.

Stir together the black-bean sauce, honey, ginger and lime juice. Add to the pan along with the reserved beef and cook, stirring often, until the vegetables are tender, about 8 minutes. Stir in the cilantro and sprinkle with sesame seeds. Spoon over the cooked pasta and serve with lime wedges and additional lime juice if desired.

TIP: For super-thin, tender slices of beef, put the steak in the freezer for 30 minutes, then remove and slice the meat across the grain.

Shrimp and Soba Noodles

Serves 4

Soba noodles are the star in this flavorful stir-fry. The nuttiness of the sauce complements the noodles. If you prefer a spicier stir-fry, simply add more of the chili-garlic paste, which can be found in the Asian-food section of most grocery stores.

1/2 cup	light coconut milk	125 mL
2 tbsp	crunchy peanut butter	30 mL
1 tbsp	grated fresh ginger	15 mL
1 tbsp	fresh lime juice	15 mL
1 tbsp	soy sauce	15 mL
1 tsp	Asian chili-garlic paste	5 mL
1/2 tsp	sesame oil	2 mL
1 tbsp	vegetable oil	15 mL
1 lb	shelled and deveined shrimp	500 g
1/2 lb	snow peas, halved on an angle	250 g
1	orange pepper, thinly sliced	1
1	red onion, halved and sliced lengthwise	1
3 cups	cooked soba noodles or whole-wheat spaghettini	750 mL
1/2 cup	grape tomatoes	125 mL
1/4 cup	chopped fresh cilantro	60 mL
	Lime wedges	

PER SERVING	
Calories	426
Fat (g)	16
Protein (g)	34
Carbohydrate (g)	40
Fiber (g)	6
Sodium (mg)	520

A very high source of fiber. An excellent source of vitamin A, vitamin C, vitamin B_6, vitamin B_{12}, folate, thiamine, iron, phosphorus and magnesium.

In a small bowl, combine the coconut milk, peanut butter, ginger, lime juice, soy sauce, chili-garlic paste and sesame oil. Stir until well combined and reserve.

Heat the vegetable oil in a wok or large skillet over medium-high heat. Add the shrimp, snow peas, orange pepper and red onion. Cook, stirring constantly, until shrimp just turns pink and vegetables are tender yet crisp, about 6 minutes. Stir in the reserved sauce and cook for 1 minute. Stir in the noodles and grape tomatoes. Cook, tossing, just until the noodles are coated and heated through. Sprinkle with fresh cilantro and toasted coconut. Serve with lime wedges.

Using Your Noodle

Pasta is a versatile ingredient that comes in all sorts of fiber-rich varieties. Pasta manufacturers are extending their lines to include whole-wheat versions of the most popular shapes, such as spaghetti, rotini, penne and macaroni. Bulk-food stores may carry lasagna and other types of noodles. For those with gluten intolerance, there are also brown-rice pastas that can be substituted for the wheat versions.

Birkenstock Spaghettini

Makes 4 main-course or 8 side-dish servings

This unusual combination will surprise everyone with its nutty, sweet flavor and contrasting textures. The sauce comes together in the time it takes you to cook the pasta.

1 lb	dry whole-wheat spaghettini	500 g
1/4 cup	green pumpkin seeds	60 mL
1/4 cup	pine nuts	60 mL
1 cup	lightly packed dried apricots	250 mL
1 tbsp	canola oil	15 mL
2 tbsp	butter	30 mL
1 cup	golden raisins	250 mL
2	shallots, minced	2
1/4 tsp	hot pepper flakes	1 mL
1 tsp	finely grated orange peel	5 mL
1/2 cup	fresh orange juice	125 mL
1/4 cup	vegetable or chicken broth	60 mL
1/2 cup	chopped fresh parsley	125 mL
1/2 tsp	each salt and freshly ground pepper (approx.)	2 mL
1/4 cup	crumbled blue cheese (optional)	60 mL

Cook the pasta according to the package directions. Meanwhile, toast the pumpkin seeds and pine nuts in a dry nonstick skillet set over medium heat for 3 minutes or until golden and fragrant. Remove from pan to a plate and reserve. Use scissors or a chef's knife to slice the apricots into thin strips.

Add the oil and butter to the skillet and return to the heat to melt the butter. Add the apricots, raisins, shallots and pepper flakes to the pan and cook, stirring, for 3 to 4 minutes or until golden and tender. Add the orange peel, juice and broth and bring to the boil. Reduce the heat to low.

Drain the pasta well and add to the skillet along with the toasted seeds, nuts, parsley, salt and pepper. Toss the pasta in the pan until well coated with the sauce. Taste and season with additional salt and pepper if desired and top with blue cheese if using.

TIP: Blue cheese is a delicious complement to the sweet dried fruit, but if you are not fond of it, substitute ¼ cup (60 mL) shaved Parmesan for an equally tasty alternative. To make the dish even more nutritious, add 2 cups (500 mL) slivered Swiss chard to the hot pasta instead of the parsley.

Oh, the Pastabilities!

Whole-wheat pasta is a terrific base for all kinds of flavors. Step out of the traditional marinara box, and try new combinations like this one, which was inspired by a fruit-and-nut mix I saw in the grocery store. What flavors do you like? Here are a few ideas for quick meals:

- Grilled chicken, vegetables and short pasta tossed with your favorite barbecue sauce and sprinkled with cheddar cheese
- Stir-fried pork, vegetables and honey-garlic sauce with spaghettini
- Tuna, olives and tomatoes in a mustard vinaigrette tossed with penne
- Green peas and mint leaves (puréed in a food processor with Parmesan and olive oil) tossed with spaghetti
- Cauliflower, chickpeas and macaroni blended with yogurt and curry paste

Oven-Dried Tomato and Spinach Penne

Serves 2

Typically, oven-drying tomatoes is an all-day process. Using small grape or cherry tomatoes will speed things up. You can dry batches of the tomatoes ahead and freeze in measured portions to toss with hot pasta.

2 cups	halved grape or cherry tomatoes	500 mL
1/4 cup	chopped fresh parsley	60 mL
3	cloves garlic, quartered	3
1/2 tsp	salt	2 mL
1/4 tsp	freshly ground pepper	1 mL
2 tbsp	olive oil	30 mL
1 tbsp	balsamic vinegar	15 mL
2 cups	uncooked whole-wheat short pasta such as penne	500 mL
2 cups	lightly packed baby spinach	500 mL

Preheat oven to 300°F (150°C). Toss the tomatoes with the parsley, garlic, salt, pepper, half the olive oil and the balsamic vinegar. Transfer the tomato mixture to a baking dish and bake for 1 to 1½ hours or until tomatoes are dark but still slightly moist.

Meanwhile, cook the pasta according to package directions. Before draining, set the spinach in the strainer and pour the hot pasta over top; drain well. Place pasta and spinach in a bowl, add the tomatoes and toss with the remaining olive oil. Season to taste with additional salt and pepper.

TIP: The longer you roast the tomatoes, the more intense the flavor will be. This recipe doubles easily for large groups.

Tomatoes

Tomatoes are a source of lycopene, a powerful antioxidant that has been linked to cancer prevention. Canned and dried tomatoes are a high source of fiber.

Sausage and Fennel Rotini

Serves 6

Caramelizing the fennel mellows the licorice flavor of this delectable vegetable. If you prefer a really spicy pasta, use hot sausages and add up to 1 tsp (5 mL) of hot pepper flakes with the fennel seed.

2 cups	dry whole-wheat rotini	500 mL
1 tbsp	olive oil	15 mL
2	Italian sausages, mild or hot	2
1 tsp	fennel seed	5 mL
1 tsp	dried thyme	5 mL
1	medium onion, thinly sliced	1
1	small bulb fennel, trimmed and thinly sliced	1
Pinch	granulated sugar	Pinch
1 tsp	each salt and freshly ground pepper	5 mL
1/2 cup	white wine or chicken broth	125 mL
1	can (28 oz/796 mL) stewed tomatoes with juice	1
1/4 cup	tomato paste	60 mL
1/4 cup	grated Parmesan cheese (optional)	60 mL

PER SERVING	
Calories	380
Fat (g)	12
Protein (g)	16
Carbohydrate (g)	55
Fiber (g)	12
Sodium (mg)	1134

A very high source of fiber. An excellent source of vitamin C, folate, niacin, thiamine, iron, phosphorus, zinc and magnesium.

Cook the pasta according to package directions, drain and keep warm. Heat olive oil in a deep nonstick skillet set over medium-high heat. Remove the casings from the sausages and crumble into the skillet. Cook, stirring often, until browned. Stir in the fennel seed and thyme and remove the sausage to a plate, leaving about 1 tbsp (15 mL) of the fat in the pan.

Return the pan to the heat and add the onion and fennel. Cook with sugar, salt and pepper, stirring often, until golden brown, about 15 minutes. Reduce the heat to medium-low, add the wine, and cook until the wine is absorbed and the fennel is tender, 5 to 10 minutes.

Stir in the tomatoes, tomato paste and sausage mixture and bring to the boil. Simmer for 5 minutes or until thickened (break the tomatoes up into large chunks with the edge of the spoon). Toss the sauce with the cooked pasta and sprinkle with Parmesan if desired.

Undercover Wonder Baked Pasta

PER SERVING	
Calories	416
Fat (g)	17
Protein (g)	32
Carbohydrate (g)	38
Fiber (g)	6
Sodium (mg)	1129

A very high source of fiber. An excellent source of vitamin A, vitamin C, vitamin E, niacin, thiamine, riboflavin, calcium, iron, phosphorus, zinc and magnesium.

Recipe Makeover: Whole-wheat pasta, loads of vegetables and a soy filling give this casserole a fiber boost that will appeal to lasagna-lovers.

Serves 8

Sneak fiber into your family's diet with this homey lasagna-inspired casserole. To make a meatless dish, substitute a "ground meat alternative" (such as TVP) and use a Parmesan-flavored soy product, which would be suitable for vegan guests.

1 lb	extra-lean ground beef	500 g
1 tbsp	vegetable oil	15 mL
1	onion, sliced	1
2	cloves garlic, minced	2
1 cup	grated zucchini	250 mL
1 cup	grated carrot	250 mL
1	green pepper, chopped	1
1½ tsp	dried thyme	7 mL
1½ tsp	dried oregano	7 mL
1½ tsp	fresh parsley	7 mL
1	jar (28 oz/796 mL) mild pasta sauce	1
1	can (28 oz/796 mL) diced tomatoes	1
¾ lb	whole-wheat spaghetti, broken into 2-inch (5 cm pieces)	350 g
1	package (10 oz/300 g) silken tofu or 2 cups (500 mL) sour cream	1
1¼ cups	grated Parmesan cheese, divided	300 mL
1 tsp	freshly ground pepper	5 mL
Pinch	ground nutmeg	Pinch

Brown the beef in a Dutch oven or large pot set over medium heat. Transfer to a paper-towel-lined strainer set over a bowl to absorb some of the fat. Heat the oil in the Dutch oven and add the onion, cooking for 5 minutes or until golden. Add the garlic, zucchini, carrot, green pepper, thyme, oregano and parsley and cook for 5 minutes longer. Stir in the pasta sauce and diced tomatoes and simmer for 10 minutes.

Meanwhile, cook the pasta according to package directions. Drain and stir into the sauce along with the ground beef.

Preheat the oven to 350°F (180°C). Blend the tofu with ¾ cup (175 mL) of the Parmesan cheese, pepper and nutmeg. Grease a 9- × 13-inch (3 L) casserole dish. Spread half the pasta mixture into the dish. Spread the tofu mixture evenly over the top. Spoon the remaining pasta mixture evenly over the tofu mixture and sprinkle with the remaining Parmesan cheese. Bake in the preheated oven for 30 minutes or until heated through and bubbly.

A Grate Idea!

Grating vegetables into pasta sauces makes them less conspicuous and more appealing for picky eaters. Try this trick with your next spaghetti sauce, or try a creamy primavera version.

Renovated Risotto

PER SERVING

Calories	416
Fat (g)	19
Protein (g)	14
Carbohydrate (g)	45
Fiber (g)	5
Sodium (mg)	997

A high source of fiber. An excellent source of vitamin A, vitamin D, niacin, thiamine, phosphorus and magnesium.

Serves 4

Okay, this isn't a pasta dish in the traditional sense, but it can be served on similar occasions. Typically, risotto is made with arborio rice, an Italian-style polished white rice. This version uses short-grain (important distinction) brown rice as its base, which offers a pleasantly nutty flavor and higher fiber content.

1 tbsp	olive oil	15 mL
2 tbsp	butter, divided	30 mL
1	onion, finely chopped	1
3/4 lb	butternut or acorn squash	350 mL
1	clove garlic, minced	1
1 cup	short-grain brown rice	250 mL
1/2 cup	white wine or chicken broth	125 mL
4 cups	chicken broth	1 L
1/3 cup	grated Parmesan cheese	75 mL
2 tbsp	chopped fresh parsley	30 mL
	Salt and freshly ground pepper	
1/4 cup	chopped pecans (optional) toasted (see Tip, page 40)	60 mL

Recipe Makeover: Simply changing from white to brown rice adds a fiber boost to this authentic Italian dish.

Heat the oil and 1 tbsp (15 mL) of the butter in a large stockpot set over medium heat. Add the onion and cook until softened and starting to brown. Peel and cut the squash into 3/4-inch (2 cm) cubes. Add the squash and garlic to the pan and cook until the squash is lightly browned at the edges, about 5 minutes.

Add the rice and stir to make sure that all the grains are coated with the oil. Add the wine and cook, stirring, until almost absorbed. Meanwhile, heat the chicken broth in a separate pot. Ladle the broth gradually into the rice, stirring constantly, allowing each ladleful to become almost absorbed before adding the next (this will take about 25 minutes). The rice will become very creamy but will stay slightly firm on the inside.

Stir in the remaining butter, Parmesan cheese and parsley and season to taste with salt and pepper. Serve immediately. Sprinkle with chopped pecans if desired.

TIP: Short-grain brown rice is essential to the creamy texture of the risotto. You can find it in your local bulk-food store.

Photo: Beef and Spinach Roulade (page 82), Smashed Potatoes, Pass Them On (page 58)

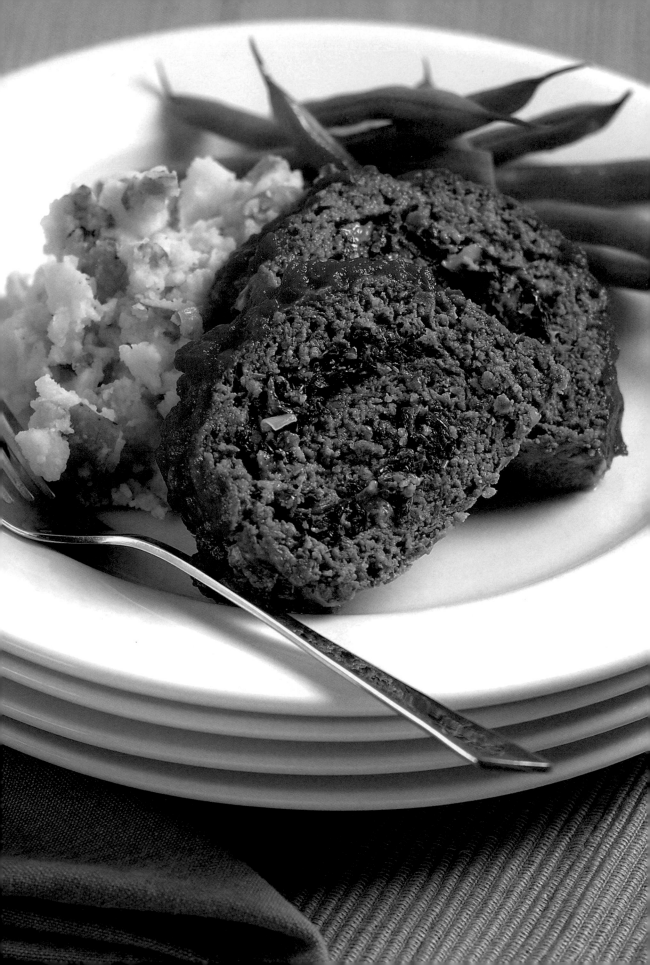

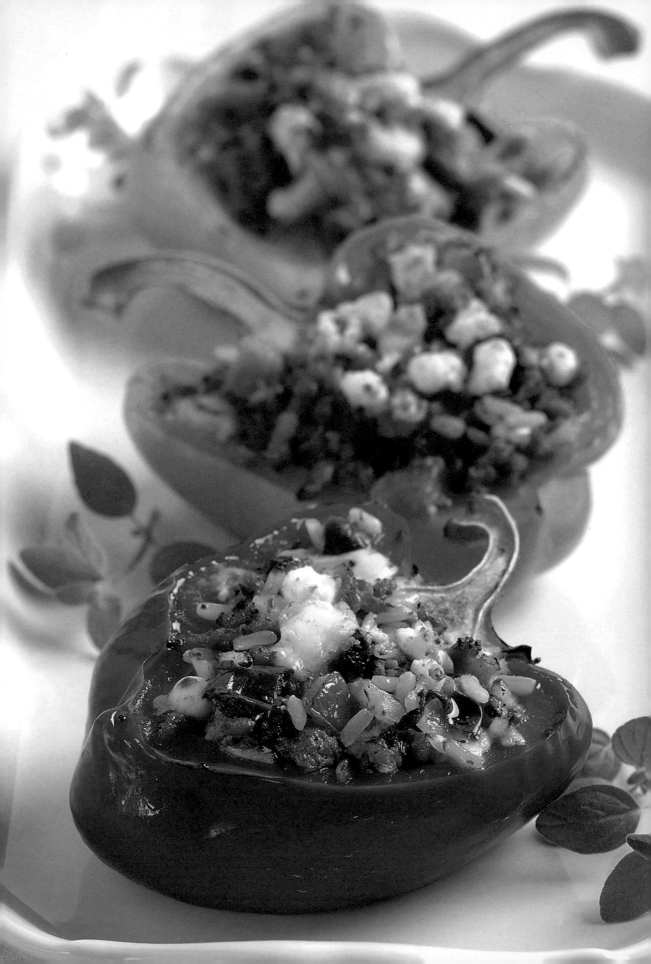

For the Meat-Lover

We are, in general, a meat-loving society, but that doesn't mean we have to throw healthy eating out with the burger wrapper. Making the choice to eat leaner meats more often, along with fiber-rich grains and vegetables adds to the variety and overall nutritional content of our diets.

Beef and Spinach Roulade

Takin' It Easy Brisket Braise

Thai Beef Haystack Sandwiches

Orchard Chèvre-Stuffed Pork Loin

Skillet Salsa Supper

Madras Ribs and Chickpeas on Couscous

Reuben Strata

Harvest Pork and Root-Vegetable Supper

Trattoria Lamb Shanks with Bean Ragout

Photo: Feta-Compli Stuffed Peppers (page 94)

Beef and Spinach Roulade

Makes 8 generous servings

Adding bran, whole-wheat breadcrumbs and a simple spinach filling increases the fiber quotient of this traditional dish. Rolling the loaf jazzes it up quickly and easily and makes it suitable for company.

Stuffing:

1 tbsp	vegetable oil	15 mL
1	small onion, chopped	1
1	clove garlic, minced	1
1	package (10 oz/300 g) frozen chopped spinach, thawed and drained	1
1 cup	fresh whole-wheat breadcrumbs	250 mL
1/2 cup	grated Parmesan cheese	125 mL

Meat Loaf:

1 lb	lean ground beef	500 g
1 tsp	dried thyme	5 mL
1/2 tsp	dried oregano	2 mL
1 tsp	salt	5 mL
1/2 tsp	freshly ground pepper	2 mL
1 cup	pasta sauce, divided	250 mL
2	eggs, beaten	2
1/4 cup	milk	60 mL
1 cup	fresh whole-wheat breadcrumbs	250 mL
1/2 cup	100% bran cereal	125 mL

Stuffing:

In a nonstick skillet, heat oil over medium heat. Add onion and cook for 2 minutes. Add garlic and cook for 2 minutes or until softened and fragrant. Cool slightly. Stir in spinach, breadcrumbs and Parmesan.

Meat Loaf:

Crumble beef into a large bowl along with thyme, oregano, salt and pepper. Stir together 1/4 cup (60 mL) of the pasta sauce, eggs, milk, breadcrumbs and bran. Combine with the meat mixture with your hands.

Preheat the oven to 375°F (190°C). Cover a rimmed cookie sheet with two layers of foil and spray the top layer with nonstick spray. Press the meat mixture into a 12- × 10-inch (30 × 25 cm) rectangle on the top layer of foil. Spread the spinach mixture evenly over the meat, leaving a 1-inch (2.5 cm) gap around the outer edges. Roll the meat jellyroll style, starting at the wide side, using the top layer of foil to help lift the meat into place and pulling the foil away as you roll the meat. Discard the used foil. Smooth the seam edge and pinch the ends closed with your fingers.

Turn seam side down on the remaining piece of foil. Bake in the preheated oven for 45 minutes. Spoon the remaining pasta sauce over the top of the roll and bake for 10 to 15 minutes more or until cooked through.

It's in the Crumbs

Meat loaves, meatballs and burgers often call for breadcrumbs to help the meat hold its shape, which offers an excellent opportunity to sneak in some fiber by using whole-wheat breadcrumbs, natural bran or crushed bran flakes.

Recipe Makeover: Adding bran flakes or whole-wheat breadcrumbs and a tasty spinach filling transforms a typical meat loaf into an elegant high-fiber dish.

Takin' It Easy Brisket Braise

PER SERVING

Calories	652
Fat (g)	35
Protein (g)	45
Carbohydrate (g)	39
Fiber (g)	8
Sodium (mg)	144

A very high source of fiber. An excellent source of vitamin A, vitamin C, vitamin B_6, vitamin B_{12}, thiamine, riboflavin, iron, phosphorus, zinc and magnesium.

Serves 6

In the tradition of a boiled supper, this is a meal in one dish that can simmer gently on the stove as you play games by a winter fire. Serve with crusty whole-wheat rolls and offer flavorful whole-grain mustards on the side.

2 tbsp	vegetable oil	30 mL
2 lb	well-trimmed beef brisket	1 kg
2 tbsp	whole-wheat or all-purpose flour	30 mL
3 cups	beef broth	750 mL
2 tbsp	brown sugar	30 mL
1 tbsp	finely grated orange peel	15 mL
1 tbsp	cider vinegar	15 mL
1	bay leaf	1
1 tsp	brown mustard seeds	5 mL
1 tsp	each salt and freshly ground pepper	5 mL
1 tsp	caraway seeds	5 mL
1	large onion, sliced	1
3	cloves garlic, sliced	3
1 lb	baby carrots	500 g
1 lb	whole baby or mini potatoes	500 g
1/2	large red cabbage	1/2

Heat the oil in a large Dutch oven set over medium-high heat. Coat the brisket with the flour and brown on each side for about 2 minutes. Gradually add the broth to the pan, scraping up any browned bits. Add the brown sugar, orange peel, vinegar, bay leaf, mustard seeds, pepper, salt and caraway to the pan, stirring to combine. Layer the sliced onion and garlic over the brisket, then add enough water to cover the meat.

Bring the pot to the boil. Reduce the heat to low and simmer, covered, for 1½ hours or until the brisket is fork-tender. Increase the heat to medium. Add the carrots and potatoes and cook, covered, for 15 minutes. Cut the cabbage into 6 wedges and nestle into the pot with the brisket, potatoes and carrots. Cook until all the vegetables are tender, about 15 minutes.

Remove the brisket from the pot, slice and transfer to a platter. With a slotted spoon, remove the vegetables and place around the sliced meat. (Save the rich broth to use as a soup base.)

Thai Beef Haystack Sandwiches

Serves 4

A healthy hoagie that comes together very quickly using lean deli-sliced beef and napa cabbage. The sauce was inspired by a traditional Thai noodle dish, but it has that "sloppy Joe" feel. If you are in a rush, substitute 4 cups (1 L) of coleslaw mix for the vegetables.

1/4 cup	rice vinegar	60 mL
1/2 cup	ketchup	125 mL
2 tbsp	fish sauce or water	30 mL
3 tbsp	light molasses	45 mL
2 tbsp	light soy sauce	30 mL
2 tbsp	fresh lemon juice	30 mL
1 tsp	granulated sugar	5 mL
1/2 tsp	chili-garlic sauce such as sambal olek or hot pepper sauce	2 mL
1 tbsp	vegetable oil	15 mL
8 oz	lean roast beef, cut into slivers	250 g
2 cups	shredded napa cabbage	500 mL
4	green onions, thinly sliced	4
1/2 cup	grated carrot	250 mL
1/4 cup	chopped fresh cilantro	60 mL
4	whole-wheat hoagie-style rolls	4

PER SERVING	
Calories	362
Fat (g)	9
Protein (g)	25
Carbohydrate (g)	49
Fiber (g)	5
Sodium (mg)	1670

A high source of fiber. An excellent source of vitamin A, vitamin C, vitamin B_6, vitamin B_{12}, folate, thiamine, iron, phosphorus, zinc and magnesium.

Recipe Makeover:
Shredded cabbage and a whole-wheat roll give a fiber boost to this Asian-influenced sloppy Joe.

In a small bowl, whisk together the vinegar, ketchup, fish sauce, molasses, soy sauce, lemon juice, sugar and chili-garlic sauce. Reserve.

Heat the oil in a large skillet set over medium-high heat. Add the roast beef, cabbage, onions and carrot and cook, stirring often, for 5 minutes. Stir in the reserved sauce and cook until cabbage is tender and the vegetable-beef mixture is well coated. Stir in the cilantro and place mixture on open hoagie rolls.

Orchard Chèvre-Stuffed Pork Loin

PER SERVING	
Calories	546
Fat (g)	30
Protein (g)	45
Carbohydrate (g)	22
Fiber (g)	3
Sodium (mg)	477

A source of fiber. An excellent source of vitamin B$_6$, vitamin B$_{12}$, niacin, phosphorus and zinc.

Serves 8

A favorite among my catering clients, this terrific stuffed roast is moist and tender. To make holiday preparation easier, make the stuffing a day ahead and get your butcher to butterfly the loin for you.

1 tbsp	butter	15 mL
1 tbsp	vegetable oil	15 mL
1	onion, diced	1
2^1/$_2$ cups	lightly packed dried fruit such as apples, pears, peaches, apricots	625 mL
1	clove garlic	1
^{1}/$_2$ cup	dry white wine	125 mL
3 lb	boneless butterflied pork loin roast	1.5 kg
1 tsp	each salt and freshly ground pepper	5 mL
4 oz	chèvre-style goat cheese	125 g
2 tbsp	Dijon mustard	30 mL
1 tbsp	maple syrup	15 mL

Heat the butter and oil together in a large, deep skillet set over medium heat. Add the onion and cook for 6 minutes or until starting to brown. Roughly chop the dried fruits and add to the pan along with the garlic. Cook, stirring often, for 2 to 3 minutes or until fruit begins to caramelize. Add the wine gradually and cook, stirring, until completely absorbed and the fruit is a rich golden brown. Remove the stuffing from the heat and cool to room temperature.

Preheat the oven to 325°F (160°C). Trim the pork of excess fat. Sprinkle the inside of the pork with salt and pepper. Spread the stuffing over the center and smooth the cheese along the center of the stuffing. Roll the pork and tie with string at 2-inch (5 cm) intervals to make a long, log-shaped roast. Set the roast seam side down on a rack in a roasting pan. Combine the mustard with the maple syrup and brush evenly over the roast. Sprinkle with additional salt and pepper if desired.

Place in the preheated oven and roast for 75 to 90 minutes or until an instant-read thermometer inserted into stuffing registers 165°F (75°C). Remove from the oven, tent with foil and let stand for 15 minutes before slicing.

Dried Fruit

Dried fruit makes an excellent fiber-rich snack and can also be an integral ingredient in baking and main-course dishes. Supermarket bulk sections are carrying more and more of these dried nuggets of gold. Dried apples, pineapples, papaya, pears, peaches, plums, cranberries, cherries, blueberries and dates are just some of the fruits available.

Skillet Salsa Supper

PER SERVING	
Calories	444
Fat (g)	20
Protein (g)	27
Carbohydrate (g)	42
Fiber (g)	7
Sodium (mg)	1314

A very high source of fiber. An excellent source of vitamin C, vitamin B$_6$, vitamin B$_{12}$, vitamin D, folate, niacin, thiamine, riboflavin, calcium, phosphorus, zinc and magnesium.

Serves 6

A family favorite, this zesty skillet dish is full of flavor, yet it comes together quickly and you'll only have one pan to wash.

1 tbsp	vegetable oil	15 mL
1	onion, chopped	1
1	green pepper, diced	1
1 1/2 cups	cubed cooked ham	375 mL
1 cup	long-grain brown rice	250 mL
1 cup	canned black beans, drained and rinsed	250 mL
1 cup	corn kernels	250 mL
1 1/2 cups	mild or medium prepared salsa	375 mL
1 1/2 cups	chicken or vegetable broth or water	375 mL
1 cup	grated cheddar cheese	250 mL
1/2 cup	crushed corn or tortilla chips (optional)	125 mL
1/4 cup	sliced green onions	60 mL
	Sour cream (optional)	

Heat the oil in a large ovenproof skillet set over medium-high heat. Add the onion, green pepper and ham and cook until vegetables are tender and the ham is lightly browned, about 5 minutes. Add the rice and stir to coat with the vegetable mixture, about 1 minute. Stir in the black beans, corn, salsa and broth and bring to a boil. Cover and reduce the heat to low. Simmer for 30 minutes or until all the liquid is absorbed and the rice is cooked.

Preheat the broiler to high. Sprinkle the cheddar over the center of the skillet; sprinkle the corn chips, if using, in a ring around the edge of the pan. Place the skillet under the preheated broiler until the cheese is bubbly, about 4 minutes. Sprinkle with green onions and serve hot with a dollop of sour cream on the side if desired.

TIP: If you don't have an ovenproof skillet, you can shield the handle of a regular pan by wrapping with foil—but only for short cooking times. You can also transfer the mixture to a casserole dish before broiling.

The Benefits of Brown

Brown rice contains about four times the amount of dietary fiber as white and has a pleasant, nutty taste. White and brown rice are essentially the same grain, except that white rice has been milled (or polished) until the bran layer is removed. The bran layer is where the fiber and essential oils are found. Brown rice can be substituted for white in any recipe—simply adjust the cooking time and the amount of fluid according to package directions.

Madras Ribs and Chickpeas on Couscous

Serves 6

A delicious new way to enjoy ribs. The ribs are fall-off-the-bone tender, and the yogurt in the Indian-influenced sauce tempers the intense curried spiciness.

2 lb	pork side ribs	1 kg
1 tsp	each salt and freshly ground pepper	5 mL
1 tbsp	vegetable oil	15 mL
1	large onion, chopped	1
2 tbsp	tomato paste	30 mL
1 tbsp	Madras-style mild or medium Indian curry paste or powder	15 mL
1	can (19 oz/540 mL) chickpeas, drained and rinsed	1
1 cup	golden raisins	250 mL
1½ cups	chicken broth	375 mL
1 cup	plain (2% or 4%) yogurt	250 mL
2 tbsp	all-purpose flour	30 mL
2 cups	cooked whole-wheat couscous or brown rice	500 mL

PER SERVING	
Calories	757
Fat (g)	20
Protein (g)	55
Carbohydrate (g)	89
Fiber (g)	8
Sodium (mg)	940

A very high source of fiber. An excellent source of vitamin B_6, vitamin B_{12}, folate, niacin, thiamine, riboflavin, iron, phosphorus, zinc and magnesium.

Preheat the oven to 350°F (180°C). Trim the ribs of excess fat and cut between the bones into individual portions. Heat the oil in a large skillet set over medium-high heat. Add the ribs in batches, browning all over. Transfer the browned ribs to a 9- × 13-inch (3 L) casserole. Reserve.

Add the onion to the pan and cook until golden, about 6 minutes. Add the tomato paste and curry paste and cook, stirring, for 1 minute. Stir in the chickpeas, raisins and chicken broth. Bring to the boil. Carefully pour the bean mixture to cover the browned ribs. Cover the casserole with foil and bake in the preheated oven for 1 to 1½ hours or until the ribs are very tender. Remove the ribs from the casserole and keep warm. Stir the yogurt and flour together until smooth and blend into the chickpeas. Return the casserole to the oven for 15 minutes or until heated through and thickened. Remove the ribs from the pan and arrange on a platter of cooked couscous or rice. Spoon the curried chickpea sauce over top and serve.

Reuben Strata

Serves 10

If you like a Reuben sandwich, you'll love this hearty strata. This is a make-ahead supper that you can prepare in the morning and just pop into the oven when you get home. Play with the kids while it bakes, then enjoy it with a crisp garden salad.

5 cups	cubed dark rye bread	1.25 L
1/2 lb	lean pastrami, cut into slivers	250 g
1 1/2 cups	well-drained sauerkraut	375 mL
2 cups	shredded Swiss cheese, divided	500 mL
8	large eggs, beaten	8
1 1/2 cups	milk	375 mL
1/4 cup	Dijon mustard	60 mL
1/4 tsp	caraway seeds (optional)	1 mL
1/4 tsp	each salt and freshly ground pepper	1 mL
	Thousand Islands dressing (optional)	

Preheat the oven to 350°F (180°C). Lightly grease a 9- × 13-inch (3 L) casserole dish. Toss the bread cubes, pastrami, sauerkraut, and 1 1/2 cups (375 mL) of the cheese in a large bowl. Turn into the prepared casserole, spreading out evenly.

Whisk the eggs with the milk, mustard, caraway seeds, salt and pepper. Pour evenly over the casserole, coating the bread with the mixture. (The casserole can be prepared up to this point and reserved in the refrigerator overnight.) Sprinkle with the remaining cheese and bake in the preheated oven for about 45 minutes or until set and golden. Let rest 10 minutes before cutting into squares. Serve with Thousand Islands dressing on the side if desired.

TIP: If using dense European-style rye bread, add 2 more large eggs to the wet mixture.

Hearty and Wholesome

Add dark, dense breads such as rye and pumpernickel to your weekly shopping list. They make excellent sandwiches with lean deli meats, taste great alongside a hearty stew and even make a delicious crumb topping in place of regular breadcrumbs. A slice of pumpernickel bread has twice as much fiber as a slice of French bread.

Harvest Pork and Root-Vegetable Supper

Serves 6

Another skillet dish! I have a busy schedule, so this is the kind of cooking I do most—all in one pan. This quick and easy supper has a lovely autumn feel.

1½ lbs	boneless pork loin chops, about 6	750 g
½ tsp	each salt and freshly ground pepper	2 mL
2	large sweet potatoes, well scrubbed	2
2	parsnips, well scrubbed	2
1 tbsp	vegetable oil	15 mL
1	onion, chopped	1
1 tbsp	chopped fresh rosemary	15 mL
1 cup	baby carrots	250 mL
1½ cups	orange or apple juice	375 mL

PER SERVING	
Calories	434
Fat (g)	22
Protein (g)	32
Carbohydrate (g)	27
Fiber (g)	4
Sodium (mg)	270

A high source of fiber. An excellent source of vitamin A, vitamin B_6, vitamin B_{12}, niacin, thiamine, riboflavin, phosphorus and zinc.

Preheat the oven to 350°F (180°C). Sprinkle the pork chops with salt and pepper. Cut the sweet potato and parsnips into 1-inch (2 cm) cubes. Heat the oil in an ovenproof skillet set over medium-high heat. Add the pork chops to the pan and cook just until browned on both sides, about 1 minute per side. Remove the chops to a plate and reserve.

Add the onion and rosemary to the pan and cook until the onion is starting to brown, about 3 minutes. Add the sweet potato and parsnip to the pan along with the carrots. Cook, stirring often, until vegetables are nicely browned. Stir in the orange juice, then nestle the pork chops into the pan. Set the pan in the preheated oven and bake for 30 to 40 minutes or until the pork is cooked through and the vegetables are tender.

TIP: If you don't have an ovenproof skillet, scrape the mixture into a 7- × 11-inch (2 L) casserole before baking.

Trattoria Lamb Shanks with Bean Ragout

Serves 6

A rustic yet elegant dish that is worth the long cooking time. Lamb shanks are an economical cut of lamb, but the flavor is delicious and worthy of special occasions. Serve with a crusty whole-wheat loaf to mop up the tasty bean ragout.

6	lamb shanks, about 4 lb (2 kg) in total	6
1/2 tsp	each salt and freshly ground pepper	2 mL
3 tbsp	whole-wheat flour	45 mL
2 tbsp	vegetable oil, divided	30 mL
2	carrots, peeled and chopped	2
1	medium onion, chopped	1
2	cloves garlic, minced	2
2 tsp	dried thyme	10 mL
1	bay leaf	1
1 tbsp	tomato paste	15 mL
1	can (28 oz/796 mL) diced tomatoes	1
1 cup	chicken broth	250 mL
1 cup	red wine	250 mL
1	can (19 oz/540 mL) navy beans	1

Sprinkle the lamb shanks with salt and pepper and coat with the flour. Heat half the oil in a large Dutch oven or skillet set over medium-high heat. Add the shanks and cook, turning often, until well browned all over. Transfer the shanks to a plate and reserve. Reduce the heat to medium and add the remaining oil, carrots, onion, garlic, thyme and bay leaf. Cook, stirring often, until the vegetables are lightly browned and fragrant, about 5 minutes.

Stir in the tomato paste and any flour left in the bowl from coating the shanks. Add the lamb, tomatoes, chicken broth and red wine. Bring the mixture to a boil. Reduce the heat to low and simmer, partially covered, for 2 hours or until lamb is very tender. (If the sauce does not cover the shanks, turn the lamb in the sauce mixture a few times to ensure even cooking.)

Remove the shanks from the pot, cover and keep warm. Stir the navy beans into the tomato mixture. Simmer, uncovered, for 10 minutes or until the beans are heated through and the sauce is reduced slightly. Use a potato masher to mash some of the beans, making the sauce thick and chunky. Spoon the ragout mixture onto a platter and top with the shanks.

TIP: A simple way to increase the fiber content of any hearty sauce is to stir in some canned beans.

Sand, Sea and Sky

Chicken and turkey are flexible dinner choices, and there are many options for them, from lean ground to speedy thighs and popular breast meats. Fish is always a healthy choice because it is high in essential fatty acids while low in total fat.

Feta-Compli Stuffed Peppers

Creamy Chicken Cobbler

Cran-Orange Stuffed Turkey Breast

Moroccan Chicken and Lentil Stew

Crunchy Flax Chicken Fingers

Pumpernickel Muffaletta

Salmon with Wild Rice and Asparagus

Sunflower-Seed-Encrusted Sole

Bombay Tuna-Stuffed Potatoes

Feta-Compli Stuffed Peppers

PER SERVING	
Calories	393
Fat (g)	17
Protein (g)	16
Carbohydrate (g)	48
Fiber (g)	5
Sodium (mg)	668

A high source of fiber. An excellent source of vitamin A, vitamin C, vitamin B$_6$, vitamin B$_{12}$, folate, riboflavin and iron.

Serves 4

A great family supper with a Mediterranean kick. Enjoy the peppers with a tossed salad and whole-wheat crusty rolls for a complete meal.

2	large red peppers, halved lengthwise and seeded	2
1/2 lb	lean ground chicken	250 g
1 tbsp	vegetable oil	15 mL
1/2 cup	chopped onion	125 mL
1	clove garlic, minced	1
1 tsp	dried oregano	5 mL
1/4 tsp	dried thyme	1 mL
1/4 tsp	each salt and freshly ground pepper	1 mL
2 tbsp	chopped black olives	15 mL
1	medium tomato, diced	1
3/4 cup	cooked barley or brown rice	175 mL
1/2 cup	crumbled feta cheese, divided	125 mL

Blanch pepper halves in boiling, salted water for 2 minutes, then set on paper towels to dry and cool. (Or cook in the microwave on high for 3 minutes.) Set, cut side up, on a rimmed baking sheet.

Set a medium-sized nonstick skillet over medium heat. Crumble in the ground chicken and cook, stirring, until well browned. Remove to a bowl. Add the oil, onion, garlic, oregano, thyme, salt and pepper to the pan and cook until onion is tender. Add the vegetables to the meat in the bowl and stir in the olives, diced tomato, barley and half the feta cheese. Stuff the mixture into the pepper halves and bake, loosely covered with foil, for 30 minutes. Uncover and sprinkle the peppers with the remaining cheese. Bake for 10 minutes more or until the peppers are tender and the cheese is melted.

Barley with Brawn

A staple food of the Roman gladiators, barley was one of the first cereals consumed. It has a pleasing nutty taste and is also a good source of soluble fiber to help lower cholesterol. Barley kernels are polished or "pearled" to remove the inedible hull. Pearl barley has less fiber than pot barley, which has more of the bran left on. (See the box on page 59 for the amount of cooking liquid and time needed to cook pearl and pot barley.)

Creamy Chicken Cobbler

Serves 6

PER SERVING	
Calories	465
Fat (g)	15
Protein (g)	40
Carbohydrate (g)	45
Fiber (g)	6
Sodium (mg)	870

A very high source of fiber. An excellent source of vitamin A, vitamin C, vitamin D, folate, thiamine and magnesium.

Use leftover chicken or pick up a rotisserie chicken from the deli to make this quick and comforting casserole. If you don't have an ovenproof skillet, transfer the mixture to an 8-cup (2 L) shallow casserole dish before topping with the crust.

1 tbsp	vegetable oil	15 mL
1	small onion, sliced	1
1	red pepper, thinly sliced	1
1	small zucchini, halved and thinly sliced	1
1 cup	sliced mushrooms (optional)	250 mL
1 tsp	dried thyme	5 mL
1/2 tsp	each salt and freshly ground pepper	2 mL
2 tbsp	all-purpose flour	30 mL
1 1/4 cups	chicken broth	300 mL
2 cups	green beans (about 1/2 lb/250 g), trimmed	500 mL
1/2 cup	sour cream	125 mL
1 tbsp	Dijon mustard	15 mL
2 cups	cooked chicken, chopped	500 mL

Cobbler Crust:

1 1/2 cups	whole-wheat flour	375 mL
1/2 cup	all-purpose flour	125 mL
2 tbsp	finely chopped parsley or green onion	30 mL
1 tbsp	granulated sugar	15 mL
1 tbsp	baking powder	15 mL
1/2 tsp	each salt and freshly ground pepper	2 mL
3 tbsp	cold cubed butter	45 mL
1 1/4 cups	buttermilk	300 mL

Recipe Makeover:
Chicken pot pie gets a fiber boost with a whole-wheat biscuit crust. It will become your new family favorite.

Preheat the oven to 375°F (190°C). In a 10-inch (25 cm) ovenproof skillet, heat the oil over medium heat. Add the onion, red pepper, zucchini and mushrooms, if using, and cook until tender, about 5 minutes, stirring occasionally.

Stir in the thyme, salt and pepper. Sprinkle the flour evenly over the skillet and stir until vegetables are coated. Gradually stir in the chicken broth and bring to the boil. Add the green beans and cook for 2 minutes. Whisk the sour cream with the mustard and stir into the vegetable mixture along with the chicken. Remove from the heat and reserve.

Cobbler Crust:
Stir together the whole-wheat flour, all-purpose flour, parsley, sugar, baking powder, salt and pepper in a large bowl. Use a pastry blender or fork to cut in the butter until crumbly, then stir in the buttermilk to make a ragged dough. Drop by large spoonfuls on top of the mixture in the

skillet, smoothing to connect the dough. Bake in the preheated oven for 30 minutes or until the biscuits are golden and cooked through.

TIP: For a crunchier topping, drop the dough by spoonfuls onto a parchment-lined cookie sheet and bake alongside the covered casserole for 20 minutes or until golden on the bottom. Transfer the biscuits to the casserole during the last 10 minutes of cooking.

Cran-Orange-Stuffed Turkey Breast

Serves 8

Simplify your holiday meals with this simple stuffed breast that makes carving a breeze. Boneless, skinless turkey can be seasonal, so you may need to order it specially from your butcher.

2 tbsp	butter	30 mL
1	small onion, chopped	1
1/2 cup	dried cranberries	125 mL
1/4 cup	golden raisins	60 mL
1 tbsp	chopped fresh rosemary or 1 tsp (5 mL) dried	15 mL
1 tbsp	finely grated orange peel	15 mL
1/2 cup	fresh orange juice	125 mL
2 cups	coarse fresh pumpernickel breadcrumbs	500 mL
1	whole boneless, skinless turkey breast or two halves, about 3 lbs (750 g) in total	1
1/2 tsp	each salt and freshly ground pepper	2 mL
1	can (14 oz/398 mL) whole-berry cranberry sauce, divided	1
2 tbsp	whole-grain Dijon mustard	30 mL
1 tbsp	brown sugar	15 mL
2 tsp	cider vinegar	10 mL

PER SERVING	
Calories	448
Fat (g)	7
Protein (g)	43
Carbohydrate (g)	54
Fiber (g)	4
Sodium (mg)	298

A high source of fiber. An excellent source of vitamin B_6, vitamin B_{12}, vitamin D, niacin, phosphorus, zinc and magnesium.

Melt the butter in a medium saucepan set over medium heat. Add the onion and cook until golden, about 3 minutes. Stir in the cranberries, raisins, rosemary and orange peel and cook 2 minutes more. Stir in the orange juice, then remove from heat. Toss with the pumpernickel crumbs and cool completely.

Preheat the oven to 325°F (160°C). Lay the turkey breast flat on a clean work surface and cut in half with a sharp knife (if necessary). Pound each half to an even thickness. Sprinkle with salt and pepper and spoon the stuffing onto one half of the breast, then top with the second half. Tie with string at 2-inch (5 cm) intervals along the width of the breast, tuck in the ends and tie one string from end to end.

In a small saucepan, whisk 3 tbsp (45 mL) of the cranberry sauce (reserve the rest for the Cran-Orange Relish—see next page), mustard, sugar and vinegar together until heated through and bubbly. Place the turkey on a rack in a roasting pan and brush with half the glaze. Bake in the preheated oven for about 1½ hours or until an instant-read thermometer inserted into the stuffing registers 180°F (83°C). While baking, brush with remaining glaze and baste with pan juices. Let stand for 10 minutes before slicing. Serve with Cran-Orange Relish if desired.

Quick Cran-Orange Relish

Coarsely chop a whole navel orange and place in a food processor. Process the orange until finely chopped. Stir with the remaining cranberry sauce and 2 tbsp (30 mL) brown sugar until well combined.

Moroccan Chicken and Lentil Stew

Serves 6

This chunky fork-and-knife stew has it all! Serve with warm whole-wheat pita wedges to complete the meal.

12	boneless, skinless chicken thighs	12
1/2 tsp	each salt and freshly ground pepper	2 mL
2 tbsp	vegetable oil	30 mL
2	small onions, quartered	2
1 lb	baby carrots	500 g
1 tsp	grated fresh ginger	5 mL
2	cloves garlic, minced	2
1 tsp	finely grated orange peel	5 mL
1 tsp	ground cumin	5 mL
1 tsp	ground coriander seed	5 mL
1 tsp	ground cinnamon	5 mL
2 tbsp	tomato paste	30 mL
1 cup	red or green lentils, rinsed and sorted	250 mL
2 cups	chicken broth	500 mL
1/4 cup	fresh orange juice	60 mL
1/4 cup	currants	60 mL
1 cup	whole prunes	250 mL
4 cups	lightly packed baby spinach	1 L
1/4 cup	sliced almonds, toasted (optional) (see Tip, next page)	60 mL
	Lemon wedges	

PER SERVING	
Calories	558
Fat (g)	17
Protein (g)	41
Carbohydrate (g)	66
Fiber (g)	12
Sodium (mg)	519

A very high source of fiber. An excellent source of vitamin A, vitamin B$_6$, vitamin E, calcium, folate, thiamine, iron, phosphorus and magnesium.

Season the chicken with salt and pepper. Heat the oil in a Dutch oven or deep skillet set over medium-high heat. Add the chicken and brown, working in batches if necessary. Transfer the browned chicken to a plate and keep warm.

Reduce the heat to medium and add onions, carrots, ginger, garlic, orange peel, cumin, coriander and cinnamon. Cook, stirring often, until vegetables are browned, about 5 minutes. Stir in the chicken, any juices that collected on the plate, tomato paste, lentils, chicken broth, orange juice, currants and prunes.

Bring the stew to the boil and simmer for 20 to 30 minutes or until the lentils are tender and most of the liquid is absorbed. Add the spinach and stir just until wilted but still bright green in color. Sprinkle with toasted almonds, if used. Serve immediately with lemon wedges and warm pitas on the side.

TIP: To toast the almonds, sprinkle them evenly into a dry skillet set over medium heat. Cook, stirring or shaking the pan often, for 3 to 5 minutes or until golden.

I Love Lentils

Lentils are the speediest legumes to cook, taking only 20 minutes. A staple in the Middle East and India, they make a great meat substitute. French or European lentils are sold with the seed coat on and maintain their shape better when cooked. Egyptian, or red, lentils are smaller and rounder. Most lentils are sold dried and can be stored in airtight containers for up to one year. Lentils are a source of calcium, vitamin A, vitamin B, iron and phosphorus.

Crunchy Flax Chicken Fingers

Serves 4

Kids love chicken fingers, and these ones contain a healthy dose of ground flax seeds, a good source of essential fatty acids. Serve with the Spicy Ketchup or your favorite condiment as a dipping sauce.

1 lb	boneless, skinless chicken breasts	500 g
1	large egg	1
2 tbsp	milk	30 mL
1¼ cups	corn flakes, crushed	300 mL
¼ cup	ground flax seeds	60 mL
3 tbsp	grated Parmesan cheese	45 mL
1 tsp	chili powder	5 mL
½ tsp	each salt and freshly ground pepper	2 mL
½ tsp	dried oregano	2 mL

Spicy Ketchup:

½ cup	ketchup	125 mL
1 tbsp	brown sugar	15 mL
1 tbsp	diced green chilies from a can	15 mL
1 tbsp	fresh lime juice	15 mL

Preheat the oven to 375°F (190°C). Trim the chicken of any fat and cut into long strips about 1 inch (2.5 cm) wide. Whisk the egg and the milk together and toss with the chicken strips. Stir together the crushed corn flakes, flax seeds, Parmesan, chili powder, salt, pepper and oregano. Pull pieces of chicken out of the egg mixture, letting the excess drip off, then coat on the crumb mixture. Set on a greased cookie sheet. Bake the strips in the preheated oven for 15 minutes or until no pink remains in the chicken. Serve with Spicy Ketchup.

Spicy Ketchup:
Combine the ketchup with the sugar, chilies and lime juice.

Focus on Flax

Flax seeds have been gaining popularity as a health food because of their high concentration of essential nutrients such as calcium, iron, niacin, phosphorus and vitamin E. They are also a source of essential omega-3 fatty acids and fiber. They have a mild nutty flavor and are best used ground in dishes so it's possible to reap all of their nutritional benefits. Store whole flax seeds in the freezer for up to 6 months.

PER SERVING (without ketchup)

Calories	353
Fat (g)	7
Protein (g)	41
Carbohydrate (g)	29
Fiber (g)	2
Sodium (mg)	674

A source of fiber. An excellent source of vitamin B_6, vitamin B_{12}, vitamin D, niacin, thiamine, riboflavin, pantothenic acid, iron and phosphorus.

Recipe Makeover:

Chicken fingers with a fiber boost of corn flakes and heart-healthy flax are quick and easy to prepare.

Pumpernickel Muffaletta

PER SERVING	
Calories	277
Fat (g)	9
Protein (g)	12
Carbohydrate (g)	38
Fiber (g)	6
Sodium (mg)	756

A very high source of fiber.
An excellent source of folate
and magnesium.

Makes 8 large portions

This super sandwich shows its beautiful layers when sliced. Make ahead and pack for cottage lunches or picnics as a meal-in-one.

1	pumpernickel round or whole-grain cottage loaf	1
1/4 cup	chopped oil-packed sun-dried tomatoes	60 mL
1/4 cup	chopped black olives	60 mL
1/2 cup	diced green pepper	125 mL
1/2 cup	chickpeas, chopped coarsely	125 mL
2 tbsp	basil pesto	30 mL
2 tbsp	mayonnaise	30 mL
4 oz	sliced lean turkey meat	125 g
6	slices light havarti or mozzarella cheese	6
2 cups	lightly packed arugula or baby spinach, washed and dried	500 mL

Cut a round cap off the top of the pumpernickel loaf. Reserve the cap. Hollow out the inside of the loaf to make a bread bowl, leaving at least 1½ inches (4 cm) of bread inside the crust. (Freeze the bread you remove to use for stuffing or breadcrumbs.)

Toss together the sun-dried tomatoes, olives, green pepper and chickpeas. Reserve. Blend the basil pesto with the mayonnaise and brush all over the interior of the loaf and the cap. Inside the bread bowl, layer half each of the turkey, cheese, sun-dried tomato mixture and arugula. Repeat the layers. Cover the filling with the reserved cap.

Wrap the loaf in plastic wrap and refrigerate for up to 24 hours. To serve, cut into wedges and secure with a toothpick.

Salmon with Wild Rice and Asparagus

Serves 4

An elegant casserole that places delicious salmon fillets atop wild rice and asparagus spears and tops them with a creamy lemon and dill sauce.

1 cup	light (5%) cream or homogenized milk	250 mL
1 tbsp	cornstarch	15 mL
1	egg, lightly beaten	1
2 tsp	finely grated lemon peel	10 mL
1 tbsp	finely chopped fresh dill or 1 tsp (5 mL) dried dill	15 mL
1/2 tsp	each salt and freshly ground pepper	2 mL
2 cups	cooked brown and wild rice blend	500 mL
3/4 lb	asparagus	350 g
4	boneless, skinless salmon fillets (each 4 to 6 oz/125 to 175 g)	4
1/2 cup	fresh whole-wheat breadcrumbs	125 mL
2 tsp	melted butter	10 mL

PER SERVING	
Calories	348
Fat (g)	11
Protein (g)	33
Carbohydrate (g)	31
Fiber (g)	3
Sodium (mg)	440

A source of fiber. An excellent source of vitamin B_6, vitamin B_{12}, vitamin D, folate, niacin, thiamine, riboflavin, phosphorus and magnesium.

Gradually whisk the cream into the cornstarch in a microwave-safe bowl. Microwave on high for 2 to 2½ minutes or until boiling and slightly thickened. (Stir at least once during the cooking.) Stir some of the hot cream into the egg, then pour the egg into the rest of the cream, stirring constantly. Microwave for 30 to 40 seconds more on high, or until thickened. Stir in the lemon peel, dill, salt and pepper. Reserve.

Preheat the oven to 350°F (180°C). Spread the rice in the bottom of a 7- × 11-inch (2 L) greased casserole dish. Blanch the asparagus in a large pot of boiling, salted water for 4 minutes. Cool in an ice-water bath and drain well. Layer the asparagus over the rice in the casserole.

Arrange the salmon on top of the asparagus and drizzle the sauce down the center of the casserole. Toss the breadcrumbs with the melted butter and sprinkle over top. Cover with foil and bake in the preheated oven for 25 minutes or until the fish flakes easily with a fork. Uncover and broil just until the breadcrumbs are toasted. Serve immediately.

TIP: Substitute asparagus with green beans, if desired.

Wild Rice Blends

As the international market opens up, the rice aisle at the supermarket is becoming more extensive. Wild rice on its own can be a little on the chewy side, but blending it with other types of rice allows for dynamic combinations of colors and textures. Long-grain white, brown, basmati, red and yellow grains are now commonly found in custom blends and pilaf mixtures.

Sunflower-Seed-Encrusted Sole

PER SERVING	
Calories	223
Fat (g)	10
Protein (g)	24
Carbohydrate (g)	10
Fiber (g)	3
Sodium (mg)	433

A source of fiber. An excellent source of vitamin B_6, vitamin B_{12}, folate, pantothenic acid, phosphorus, zinc and magnesium.

Recipe Makeover: This whole-wheat crumb and seed crust provides a delicious fiber boost over traditionally greasy battered fish!

Serves 4

Try this simple yet appetizing encrusted sole for a healthy weeknight supper, accompanied by a tossed green salad.

4	sole fillets, fresh or thawed if frozen	4
	(each 4 to 6 oz /125 to 175 g)	
1/2 tsp	each salt and freshly ground pepper	2 mL
1 tbsp	fresh lemon juice	15 mL
1/4 cup	wheat germ	60 mL
1/4 cup	fresh whole-wheat breadcrumbs	60 mL
1/2 cup	unsalted sunflower seeds	125 mL
2 tbsp	extra-virgin olive oil, divided	30 mL
2 tbsp	minced fresh parsley	30 mL
1 tbsp	whole-grain Dijon mustard	15 mL
	Lemon wedges	

Preheat the oven to 425°F (220°C). Lay the sole fillets out on a parchment-lined baking sheet. Sprinkle with salt and pepper and drizzle with the lemon juice. Blend together the wheat germ, breadcrumbs, sunflower seeds, half the olive oil, parsley and mustard.

Press one-quarter of the crumb mixture onto the top of each fillet. Drizzle each fillet with the remaining oil. Bake in the preheated oven for about 10 minutes. Turn the broiler to high and broil for 2 minutes or until cooked through and the topping is lightly browned. Serve with lemon wedges.

Bombay Tuna-Stuffed Potatoes

Serves 4 to 8

These savory stuffed potatoes are excellent served with a leafy green salad and perfect to keep in the freezer for quick meals. Leave out the tuna and substitute chicken, chickpeas or extra vegetables for a variation.

4	large baking potatoes, about 2 lb (1 kg) in total	4
1/2 cup	plain 2% yogurt	125 mL
1/4 cup	light mayonnaise	60 mL
1 tbsp	fresh lime juice	15 mL
1 tsp	mild Indian-style curry paste or powder	5 mL
2	cans (each 6 oz/175 g) chunk tuna, drained	2
2 cups	chopped broccoli	500 mL
1/4 cup	chopped green onion	60 mL
1/2 cup	diced red pepper	125 mL
1/2 cup	grated cheddar cheese (light if possible)	125 mL
1/4 cup	crushed bran flakes	60 mL

PER SERVING (1 whole potato)	
Calories	563
Fat (g)	10
Protein (g)	43
Carbohydrate (g)	80
Fiber (g)	13
Sodium (mg)	582

A very high source of fiber. An excellent source of vitamin A, vitamin B_6, vitamin B_{12}, vitamin C, vitamin E, folate, niacin, thiamine, riboflavin, pantothenic acid, calcium, iron, phosphorus, zinc and magnesium.

Pierce the potatoes with a fork. Bake in a 350°F (180°C) oven for about 1 hour or until fork-tender (or in the microwave on high for 10 to 15 minutes). Cool until easy to handle, then cut each in half. Using a spoon, scoop most of the cooked potato into a bowl, leaving about a 1/2-inch (1 cm) rim for stability. Set the shells on a baking sheet.

Stir the yogurt with the mayonnaise, lime juice and curry paste. Combine the potato flesh, with the tuna, broccoli, green onion, red pepper and yogurt mixture, stirring until well blended. Spoon the filling back into the shells (they will be well rounded). Sprinkle with cheddar cheese and the crushed bran flakes. (The potatoes can be prepared up to this point and frozen in airtight containers for up to 1 month or held in the refrigerator for 1 day.) Return the stuffed potatoes to the oven and bake for 30 minutes. (Bake for 40 minutes from frozen.)

Easy Bakes

Whether to keep on hand for snacking or special occasions, a store of healthful baked goods is always useful. Control the fat and fiber content by making these quick breads and goodies from scratch.

Gemstone Soda Bread

PER SERVING (2 slices)	
Calories	306
Fat (g)	5
Protein (g)	10
Carbohydrate (g)	59
Fiber (g)	6
Sodium (mg)	567

A very high source of fiber. An excellent source of vitamin D and thiamine.

Makes 1 large loaf, about 20 slices

Bejeweled with plenty of dried fruit, this rustic loaf is delicious served as a snack with tea or with a main-course dish such as the Moroccan Chicken and Lentil Stew on page 97.

3 cups	whole-wheat flour	750 mL
1½ cups	all-purpose flour (approx.)	375 mL
1 cup	chopped dried apricots	250 mL
½ cup	dried cranberries	125 mL
¼ cup	dried blueberries or raisins	60 mL
3 tbsp	granulated sugar	45 mL
1½ tsp	baking powder	7 mL
1½ tsp	baking soda	7 mL
1 tsp	salt	5 mL
3 tbsp	cold butter, cubed	45 mL
2¼ cups	buttermilk	550 mL

Preheat the oven to 375°F (190°C). Combine the whole-wheat flour, all-purpose flour, apricots, cranberries, blueberries, sugar, baking powder, baking soda and salt in a large bowl and mix well. Cut in butter until crumbly, using a pasty blender or two knives. Make a well in the dry ingredients and, using a fork, stir in buttermilk just until a ragged dough forms.

Turn the dough out onto a lightly floured surface and gather into a ball. Knead lightly about 10 times or until no dry patches remain. Place the dough on a parchment-paper-lined baking sheet and pat into a 2-inch (5 cm) thick disk.

Dust the top of the loaf generously with all-purpose flour and score with a large X, 1 inch (2.5 cm) deep, with a sharp knife. Bake in the preheated oven for 40 to 45 minutes or until golden and a tester inserted in center comes out clean.

TIP: For different flavors, try substituting other dried fruit (chopping any large pieces). This bread freezes well, so you can store unused portions, tightly bagged, in the freezer for up to 1 month. You could also divide the dough into two loaves and freeze one of them for another time. Just decrease the baking time by 10 minutes.

Cast-Iron Cornbread

Serves 6

Crunchy on the outside, golden and tender on the inside, cornbread made in a cast-iron skillet is the best you'll ever taste.

1 tbsp	vegetable oil	15 mL
1½ cups	finely ground cornmeal	375 mL
½ cup	whole-wheat flour	125 mL
3 tbsp	granulated sugar	45 mL
1 tbsp	baking powder	15 mL
1 tsp	baking soda	5 mL
¾ tsp	salt	4 mL
½ cup	corn kernels	125 mL
¼ cup	finely chopped pimento	60 mL
2 tbsp	diced green chilies from a can	30 mL
1½ cups	buttermilk	375 mL
3	eggs, lightly beaten	3
3 tbsp	melted butter	45 mL

PER SERVING	
Calories	351
Fat (g)	12
Protein (g)	10
Carbohydrate (g)	51
Fiber (g)	3
Sodium (mg)	828

A source of fiber. An excellent source of vitamin D and folate.

Grease a 10-inch (25 cm) cast-iron skillet with vegetable oil and place on the center rack of your oven. Preheat oven and skillet to 400°F (200°C). In a medium bowl, stir together the cornmeal, flour, sugar, baking powder, baking soda and salt. Stir in corn, pimento and chilies until well coated. In a separate bowl, whisk together buttermilk, eggs and butter until combined. Stir into cornmeal mixture and mix just until moistened.

Remove the skillet from the oven and immediately pour the batter in (it will sizzle). Return the pan to the oven and bake for 20 to 22 minutes or until browned on top and a toothpick inserted in the center comes out clean. Serve warm.

A-maize-ing!

In North America, corn is most often eaten as a vegetable—corn on the cob is a staple at any summer barbecue. Yet corn is actually a grain and deserves the acclaim that this status can bring. Corn flour and cornmeal are used extensively in African countries as a food staple. Cornmeal can be used to line pizza pans and cooked in tortillas, muffins and porridge.

Cornmeal is also the basis of polenta, a northern Italian dish that can be served warm or cool, topped with sauce or grilled. A basic recipe consists of 1 part coarse cornmeal and 2 parts water or broth. Gradually stir the cornmeal into the water and bring to the boil. Reduce the heat and simmer, stirring often, for about 30 minutes or until the cornmeal loses its gritty texture. At this point, it can be mounded on a platter or poured into a greased pan to be cut into shapes and baked, grilled or fried. You can also buy polenta in tubes in the deli section of many grocery stores. Try slicing it and baking it topped with your favorite pasta sauce and cheese.

Savory Garlic and Herb Spelt Biscuits

Makes 18 biscuits

Finding spelt flour may mean a search through your supermarket's organic or natural-foods section or even a trip to a health-food store, but the nutritional benefits of spelt are worth it. This easy recipe is a great introduction to a fiber-rich grain.

2¼ cups	spelt flour or whole-wheat cake and pastry flour	550 mL
2½ tsp	baking powder	12 mL
1 tbsp	finely chopped fresh rosemary	15 mL
1 tbsp	finely chopped fresh parsley	15 mL
1 tbsp	finely chopped fresh chives	15 mL
1 tbsp	dried minced garlic	15 mL
¾ tsp	salt	4 mL
½ tsp	freshly ground pepper	2 mL
½ tsp	baking soda	2 mL
⅓ cup	cold butter, cubed	75 mL
1 cup	buttermilk	250 mL

PER SERVING (2 biscuits)	
Calories	175
Fat (g)	8
Protein (g)	5
Carbohydrate (g)	23
Fiber (g)	4
Sodium (mg)	712

A high source of fiber. An excellent source of vitamin D.

Preheat the oven to 400°F (200°C). Stir the flour with the baking powder, rosemary, parsley, chives, garlic, salt, pepper, baking soda and butter. Combine with a pastry blender or fork until the mixture resembles coarse crumbs. Add the buttermilk and stir the mixture with a fork until it forms a ragged dough.

Turn the dough out onto a clean, lightly floured surface. Knead gently 10 times and pat into a ½-inch (1 cm) thick round. (If the dough is sticky, coat your hands with flour for easy handling.) Cut 2-inch (5 cm) rounds with a cookie cutter or the rim of a glass. Set the rounds on an ungreased baking sheet. Press the scraps together to form additional rounds.

Bake in the preheated oven for 12 to 15 minutes or until golden on the bottom. Cool on the pan on racks. If you are not using the biscuits right away, freeze them between layers of waxed paper in an airtight container and warm gently in the oven before serving.

TIP: Spelt flour requires less leavening agent than wheat flour; if substituting whole-wheat flour, increase the amount of baking powder to 1 tbsp (15 mL).

Spelt

Spelt is an ancient cereal grain that is gaining popularity in North America. It is high in protein and fiber and is often tolerated by those with wheat allergies. It has a pleasant nutty flavor and can be substituted for wheat flour in most recipes, although you may need to reduce the liquid by one-quarter to achieve optimum results. Buy it in the organic section of your supermarket or in bulk- or health-food stores.

Photo: Gemstone Soda Bread
(page 108),
Orange-Chocolate Fig Spread
(page 19)

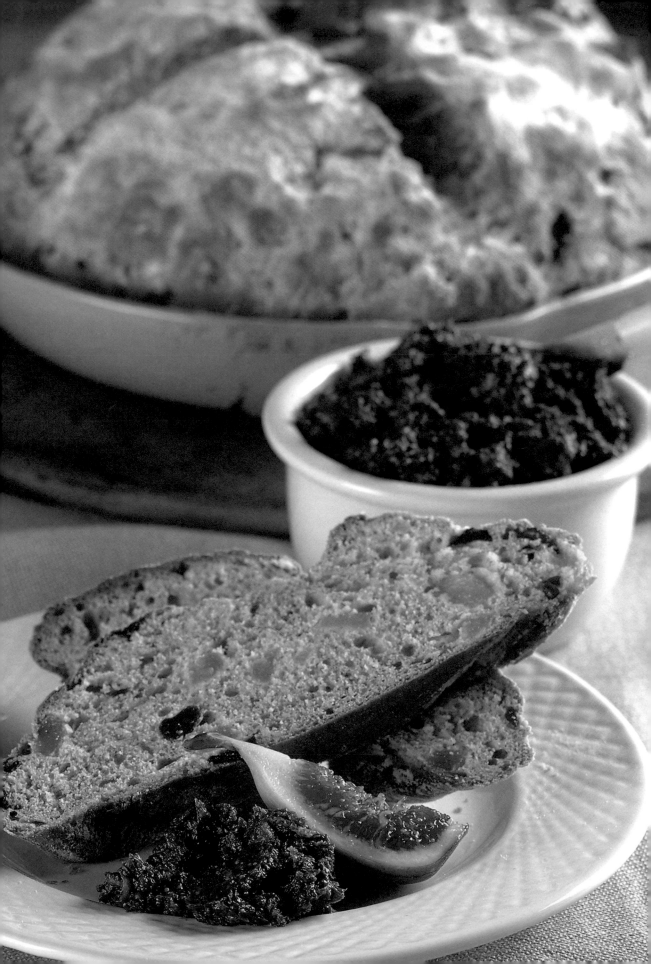

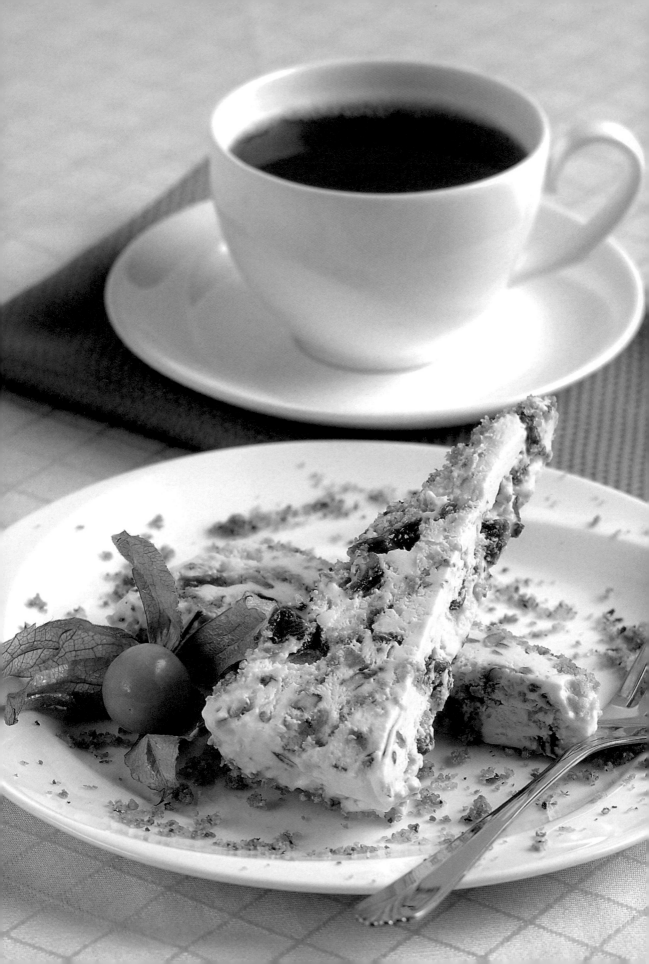

Caramel-Apple Sticky Buns

Makes 12 buns

Cinnfully delicious! For a heavenly brunch treat, try these fiber-enhanced sticky buns. Using quick-rising yeast cuts the preparation time in half and makes the buns easier for a weekend treat.

Dough:

2 cups	whole-wheat flour	500 mL
1 cup	all-purpose flour (approx.)	250 mL
1 cup	natural wheat bran	250 mL
1/4 cup	granulated sugar	60 mL
2	packages (each 1/4 oz/7 g) quick-rising yeast	2
1/2 tsp	salt	2 mL
1/4 cup	butter	60 mL
3/4 cup	milk	175 mL
1/2 cup	water	125 mL
1	egg, beaten	1

Topping:

1 cup	lightly packed brown sugar	250 mL
1/4 cup	corn syrup	60 mL
1/4 cup	light (5%) cream	60 mL
2 tbsp	butter	30 mL

Filling:

1/4 cup	lightly packed brown sugar	60 mL
1 tbsp	ground cinnamon	15 mL
1 cup	coarsely chopped pecans	250 mL
1 cup	chopped dried apple	250 mL
2 tbsp	melted butter	30 mL

PER SERVING (1 bun)	
Calories	523
Fat (g)	16
Protein (g)	8
Carbohydrate (g)	96
Fiber (g)	11
Sodium (mg)	253

A very high source of fiber. An excellent source of vitamin D, folate, thiamine, iron and magnesium.

Recipe Makeover:

Typically full of fat and simple carbs, sticky buns get a fiber boost from the tender whole-wheat dough and the savory dried-apple filling.

Dough:

Combine the flours, bran, sugar and yeast in a large bowl and stir to combine. In a small saucepan, heat the salt, butter, milk and water just until the butter is melted. Make a well in the dry ingredients and pour in the warm milk and the beaten egg. Use a fork to stir until the mixture forms a ragged dough. Gather the mixture together into a ball.

Transfer the dough to a lightly floured board and knead for about 6 minutes or until smooth and elastic, adding more flour if necessary to keep it from sticking to your hands. Transfer to a greased bowl and let stand in a warm place for 15 minutes. Preheat the oven to 375°F (190°C) and prepare the topping and filling. (See the next page).

Photo: Bread Pudding Semi-Freddo (page 130)

Topping:
Combine the brown sugar, corn syrup, cream and butter in a heavy saucepan and bring to the boil over medium heat. Remove from heat and pour evenly into a greased 9- × 13-inch (3 L) baking dish.

Filling:
Combine brown sugar, cinnamon, pecans and apple.

Roll the rested dough into an 18- × 14-inch (45 × 35 cm) rectangle. Brush with the melted butter, leaving a 1-inch (2.5 cm) border around the edge. Sprinkle the apple mixture over the buttered portion. Starting at the short end, roll up tightly and pinch at the seam to seal. Cut with a serrated knife into 12 pieces and place, cut side down, in the prepared pan. Bake in the preheated oven for 25 minutes or until golden and the top sounds hollow when tapped. Let stand in the pan for 5 minutes. Invert onto a serving platter, scraping off any remaining filling in the pan to drizzle over the buns.

High Fiber

Take away some of the guilt of indulging in sweet snacks by adding more fiber and therefore increasing the nutritional value. In most baked recipes, up to three-quarters of the white flour can be replaced with whole-wheat.

Mahogany Spice Loaf

Makes 1 loaf, 12 slices

This moist and delicious loaf has a surprising ingredient: a can of baked beans! Try it, and you'll be pleasantly surprised by this low-fat quick bread.

1 cup	all-purpose flour	250 mL
3/4 cup	whole-wheat flour	175 mL
2 tsp	baking powder	10 mL
1 tsp	baking soda	5 mL
2 tsp	ground ginger	10 mL
1 tbsp	ground cinnamon	15 mL
1/2 tsp	ground allspice	2 mL
1/4 tsp	salt	1 mL
1	can (14 oz/398 mL) vegetarian baked beans in tomato sauce	1
1 cup	tightly packed dark brown sugar	250 mL
1/4 cup	canola oil	60 mL
2	eggs	2
1 tsp	vanilla	5 mL

Topping:

1/4 cup	chopped pecans or walnuts	60 mL
1 tbsp	maple syrup	15 mL

PER SERVING (1 slice)	
Calories	240
Fat (g)	7
Protein (g)	5
Carbohydrate (g)	41
Fiber (g)	4
Sodium (mg)	358

A high source of fiber. An excellent source of vitamin D.

Lightly grease a 9- × 5-inch (2 L) loaf pan and set aside. Preheat the oven to 350°F (180°C). In a large bowl, combine the all-purpose flour, whole-wheat flour, baking powder, baking soda, ginger, cinnamon, allspice and salt. Use a whisk to blend all the dry ingredients together.

In a food processor or blender, combine beans, sugar, oil, eggs and vanilla. Process the mixture until smooth. Make a well in the dry ingredients and pour in the bean mixture. Stir with a wooden spoon just until moistened. Scrape into the prepared pan. Combine the pecans with the maple syrup and spoon down the center of the batter. Bake the loaf in the preheated oven for 45 minutes or until a toothpick inserted in the center comes out clean. Cool on a wire rack.

Sweet Substitution

One of the ways to lower the fat content of quick breads such as muffins and loaves is to substitute puréed fruit for some of the oil. Taking this further, we substituted puréed baked beans for the typical applesauce, crushed pineapple or prunes.

Palm Grove Loaf

Makes 1 loaf, 12 slices

Shredded coconut, pecans and dates star in this delicious tea-time loaf. You may want to double this recipe because it won't last long.

3/4 cup	finely chopped dates	175 mL
3/4 cup	quick-cooking rolled oats	175 mL
1 1/2 cups	boiling water	375 mL
1/3 cup	softened butter	75 mL
2	eggs	2
3/4 cup	lightly packed brown sugar	175 mL
1 tsp	vanilla	5 mL
1/2 tsp	salt	2 mL
1 cup	whole-wheat flour	250 mL
1/2 cup	all-purpose flour	125 mL
1 tsp	baking soda	5 mL
1 tsp	ground cinnamon	5 mL

Coconut Layer:

1/3 cup	shredded unsweetened coconut	125 mL
1/3 cup	chopped pecans	125 mL
2 tbsp	brown sugar	30 mL

Preheat the oven to 350°F (180°C). Stir the dates and oats with the boiling water. Stir in the butter until melted, and cool the mixture to room temperature. In a separate bowl, whisk the eggs with the sugar, vanilla and salt. Stir in date-oat mixture.

Combine the flours, baking soda and cinnamon. Stir with a whisk, then add to the wet ingredients, stirring with a wooden spoon until well combined.

Coconut Layer:
Combine the coconut with the pecans and brown sugar. Reserve.

Grease a 9- × 5-inch (2 L) loaf pan. Spoon half the loaf batter into the pan. Sprinkle with half the coconut mixture. Spoon the rest of the batter over top and sprinkle with the remaining coconut mixture. Bake in the preheated oven for 1 hour or until a toothpick inserted in the center of the loaf comes out clean.

Kitchen Sink Cookies

Makes about 4 dozen cookies

With three simple variations, you can change the flavor of this cookie to suit any sweet tooth. Or you can make up your own variations using 2 cups (500 mL) of your favorite dried fruits and nuts.

1 cup	whole-wheat flour	250 mL
1 cup	all-purpose flour	250 mL
1/2 cup	quick-cooking rolled oats	125 mL
1 tsp	baking powder	5 mL
1/4 tsp	baking soda	1 mL
1/2 tsp	salt	2 mL
2/3 cup	softened butter	150 mL
2/3 cup	lightly packed brown sugar	150 mL
2	eggs	2
2 tbsp	milk	30 mL
1 tsp	vanilla	5 mL

Preheat the oven to 375°F (190°C). Use a whisk to stir together the whole-wheat flour, all-purpose flour, oats, baking powder, baking soda and salt in a medium bowl. In a separate bowl, beat the butter and brown sugar with an electric mixer until light and fluffy. Beat in the eggs one at a time. Beat in the milk and vanilla.

With the mixer on low or using a wooden spoon, blend in the dry ingredients. Fold in fruit and nuts from the variations below. Drop by heaping teaspoons onto parchment-lined cookie sheets. Bake in the preheated oven for 8 to 10 minutes or until lightly browned.

Variations:

Tropical Island Cookies: Add 1 tsp (5 mL) ground ginger to the dry mixture and stir in 1 cup (250 mL) diced dried pineapple, 1/2 cup (125 mL) flaked sweetened coconut and 1/2 cup (125 mL) chopped cashews.

Chocolate Cherry Pecan Cookies: Replace 1/2 cup (125 mL) of the all-purpose flour with unsweetened cocoa powder and stir in 1 1/2 cups (375 mL) pecans and 1/2 cup (125 mL) dried sour cherries or cranberries.

Lemon Blueberry Almond Cookies: Add 1 tbsp (15 mL) finely grated lemon rind along with the vanilla and stir in 1 1/2 cups (375 mL) toasted slivered almonds and 1/2 cup (125 mL) dried blueberries.

TROPICAL ISLAND COOKIES PER SERVING (2 cookies)

Calories	155
Fat (g)	8
Protein (g)	3
Carbohydrate (g)	20
Fiber (g)	2
Sodium (mg)	141

A source of fiber. An excellent source of vitamin D.

CHOCOLATE CHERRY PECAN COOKIES PER SERVING (2 cookies)

Calories	166
Fat (g)	11
Protein (g)	3
Carbohydrate (g)	17
Fiber (g)	2
Sodium (mg)	136

A source of fiber. An excellent source of vitamin D.

LEMON BLUEBERRY ALMOND COOKIES PER SERVING (2 cookies)

Calories	181
Fat (g)	10
Protein (g)	4
Carbohydrate (g)	19
Fiber (g)	2
Sodium (mg)	139

A source of fiber. An excellent source of vitamin D.

Recipe Makeover: A fiber boost of whole-wheat flour, oats, dried fruit and nuts makes these cookies a healthy treat.

Pineapple-Cherry Upside-Down Cake

PER SERVING	
Calories	330
Fat (g)	14
Protein (g)	5
Carbohydrate (g)	48
Fiber (g)	2
Sodium (mg)	386

A source of fiber. An excellent source of vitamin D.

Serves 10

With a caramelized golden topping and tart sour cherries, this whole-wheat-enhanced cake is so delicious and pretty, you'll forget it is good for you.

Topping:

1	can (14 oz/398 mL) pineapple chunks	1
3 tbsp	melted butter	45 mL
1/4 cup	granulated sugar	60 mL
1/2 cup	dried sour cherries or cranberries	125 mL

Cake:

1/2 cup	softened butter	125 mL
3/4 cup	granulated sugar	175 mL
2	eggs	2
1 tsp	vanilla	5 mL
3/4 cup	all-purpose flour	175 mL
3/4 cup	whole-wheat flour	175 mL
1 tsp	baking soda	5 mL
1 tsp	baking powder	5 mL
1/4 tsp	salt	1 mL
1 cup	buttermilk	250 mL

Topping:

Drain the pineapple well and dry on pieces of paper towel. Melt the butter in a nonstick skillet set over medium heat. Sprinkle the sugar evenly over the top and stir until dissolved. Place the pineapple chunks in the pan in a single layer and cook, turning often, until golden brown, about 8 minutes. Stir in the cherries and remove the pan from the heat. Spoon the mixture into the bottom of a greased 10-inch (3 L) Bundt pan.

Cake:

Preheat the oven to 350°F (180°C). Beat the butter with the sugar until fluffy. Add the eggs and vanilla and beat until smooth. In a separate bowl, whisk together flours, baking soda, baking powder and salt. Combine with butter mixture in two additions, alternating with the buttermilk and mixing well between additions. Bake the cake in the preheated oven for 45 minutes or until the top springs back when lightly touched. Cool in pan on a rack for 15 minutes, then invert onto a serving platter.

TIP: If you don't have buttermilk handy, stir 1 tbsp (15 mL) of lemon juice into 1 cup (250 mL) of milk.

Show-Stopping Sweet Endings

You can have your cake and eat it too with these decadent yet healthful desserts.

Mixed Berry Crunch Trifle

Serves 8

Very pretty with its layers of dark red on white, this upscale version of a fruit crisp is perfect for special occasions. Each component can be made ahead and the trifle assembled shortly before you want to use it.

Oatmeal Crunch Layer:

1¹/₂ cups	quick-cooking rolled oats (not instant)	375 mL
¹/₂ cup	whole-wheat flour	125 mL
¹/₂ cup	lightly packed brown sugar	125 mL
¹/₄ cup	sliced or slivered almonds	60 mL
¹/₃ cup	softened butter	75 mL

Mixed Berry Filling:

5 cups	frozen mixed berries such as cranberries, strawberries, blueberries, raspberries	1.25 L
¹/₂ cup	granulated sugar	125 mL
1 tbsp	cornstarch	15 mL
1 tbsp	cold water	15 mL
2 tbsp	orange liqueur such as Grand Marnier (optional)	30 mL

Cinnamon Cream:

1³/₄ cup	smooth light ricotta cheese	425 g
2 tbsp	brown sugar	30 mL
1 tsp	ground cinnamon	5 mL
1 tsp	vanilla	5 mL

Oatmeal Crunch Layer:

Preheat the oven to 350°F (180°C). Stir together the oats, flour, brown sugar and almonds in a large bowl. Using a pastry blender or two knives, cut the butter into the mixture until it resembles granola. Evenly press the mixture onto a rimmed baking sheet lined with foil (for easy cleanup). Bake for 15 to 18 minutes in the preheated oven. Cool the mixture and use your fingers to crumble it. Store the oatmeal crunch in an airtight container for up to 1 week. (This also makes a great topping for fresh fruit and yogurt.)

Mixed Berry Filling:

Combine the frozen fruit and sugar in a large saucepan set over medium heat. Bring the fruit to the boil, turn the heat to low and simmer for 5 minutes or until the fruit is tender. Blend the cornstarch into the cold water until smooth and then into the fruit mixture. Cook, stirring, for 2 minutes or until mixture thickens. Cool to room temperature. Don't worry if the mixture is still a bit liquid—it will thicken more as it cools.

Store it in the refrigerator until ready to use (up to 1 week) or in the freezer to have handy at any time.

Cinnamon Cream:
Simply blend the ricotta with the brown sugar, cinnamon and vanilla until smooth, using a spatula. Store the mixture in the refrigerator until ready to use (up to 3 days).

To assemble:
So that the topping stays crunchy and delicious, assemble the trifle within 30 minutes of serving. Start by layering a third of the crunch mixture in a trifle dish or a pretty glass bowl. Top with half the fruit mixture, then add half the cream. Repeat layers once and top with the remaining crumb mixture.

For a Summer Variation:
Replace the frozen fruit with fresh berries, and leave out the cornstarch and water. Simply macerate the fresh berries in the sugar and liqueur for up to 1 day before assembling. Replace the brown sugar in the ricotta filling with icing sugar and, to complement the fresh flavors, add 1 tbsp (15 mL) finely grated orange peel instead of the cinnamon.

Berry Delicious

Eating berries on a regular basis may help to protect against the damage caused by free radicals, agents that damage your body's cells. Berries, such as cranberries, blackberries and black currants, contain antioxidants that can boost protection against diseases such as heart disease and cancer. The bountiful seeds found in most berries make them very high sources of fiber.

Diablo Pudding Cake with Spiked Sour-Cherry Sauce

Serves 12

PER SERVING	
Calories	424
Fat (g)	6
Protein (g)	4
Carbohydrate (g)	97
Fiber (g)	9
Sodium (mg)	563

A very high source of fiber.
An excellent source of
vitamin D.

This decadent chocolate pudding cake gets its delicious moistness from high-fiber dates. The Kahlua-enhanced sour-cherry sauce provides a delicious finishing touch. This dessert sounds much more complicated than it is.

Diablo Pudding Cake:

2¹/₂ cups	coarsely chopped dates	625 mL
1³/₄ cups	strong coffee	425 mL
4 tsp	baking soda	20 mL
³/₄ cup	all-purpose flour	175 mL
³/₄ cup	whole-wheat flour	175 mL
¹/₂ cup	unsweetened cocoa powder	125 mL
1 tbsp	baking powder	15 mL
1 tsp	ground cinnamon	5 mL
¹/₃ cup	softened butter	75 mL
1¹/₃ cups	granulated sugar	325 mL
3	eggs	3
1 tsp	vanilla	5 mL

Spiked Sour-Cherry Sauce:

2 cups	frozen and thawed or canned sour cherries	500 mL
¹/₂ cup	lightly packed brown sugar	125 mL
1 tbsp	cornstarch	15 mL
2 tbsp	Kahlua (optional)	30 mL
	Whipped cream (optional)	

Diablo Pudding Cake:
Preheat the oven to 325°F (160°C). Place the dates and coffee in a saucepan set over medium heat. Cover and bring to the boil. Remove the lid and simmer for 5 minutes, stirring occasionally. Remove the saucepan from the heat and stir in the baking soda. Let stand for 15 minutes.

Grease 12 ramekins or custard cups. Stir the all-purpose flour with the whole-wheat flour, cocoa powder, baking powder and cinnamon. Reserve. Beat the butter with the sugar in a large bowl until fluffy. Add the eggs, one at a time, beating well between additions and scraping down the sides of the bowl with a spatula as needed. Stir in the vanilla. Gradually beat in the flour mixture until combined. Stir in the dates until well blended. Spoon into the prepared ramekins, to about three-quarters full. Smooth the tops flat.

Place the puddings in a deep roasting pan. Add boiling water to the pan until it comes halfway up the sides of the puddings. Cover the pan with foil, making 6 vent holes in it to allow the steam to escape. Bake in the preheated oven for 60 minutes or until a cake tester inserted in the center of one pudding comes out with just a few moist crumbs attached. Remove the puddings from the water. Turn out of the ramekins and serve immediately with the Spiked Sour-Cherry Sauce and whipped cream, if desired, or reserve and reheat later in the microwave.

Spiked Sour-Cherry Sauce:
Drain the cherries but reserve ¼ cup (60 mL) of the juice. Combine the cherries with the brown sugar in a saucepan set over medium heat. Stir the reserved juices with the cornstarch, then stir into the cherries. Bring the mixture to the boil. Reduce the heat and cook until thickened, about 3 minutes. Remove the pan from the heat and stir in the Kahlua if using. Serve warm with the puddings. (If making the sauce ahead, reheat gently on the stovetop before serving.)

Carrot-Pineapple Tower Cake

Serves 12

This decadent mile-high cake is much like the traditional one, but it has an additional fiber kick from the whole-wheat flour.

³/₄ cup	vegetable oil	175 mL
³/₄ cup	granulated sugar	175 mL
3	eggs	3
1	can (19 oz/540 mL) crushed pineapple, drained well	1
2 cups	lightly packed grated carrots	500 mL
¹/₂ cup	raisins	125 mL
1 cup	whole-wheat flour	250 mL
³/₄ cup	all-purpose flour	175 mL
2 tsp	ground cinnamon	10 mL
1¹/₂ tsp	baking powder	7 mL
1¹/₂ tsp	baking soda	7 mL
¹/₂ tsp	ground allspice	2 mL

Cream Cheese Frosting:

8 oz	brick-style cream cheese, softened	250 g
¹/₄ cup	softened butter	60 mL
4 cups	icing sugar	1 L
²/₃ cup	orange marmalade (optional)	150 mL

Preheat the oven to 325°F (160°C). Grease three 8-inch (20 cm) round cake pans and line each one with a square of parchment paper. Using an electric mixer, beat the oil with the sugar until fluffy. Beat in the eggs one at a time until the mixture is light and thickened. Reduce the speed and stir in the crushed pineapple, carrots and raisins.

In a separate bowl, stir the whole-wheat flour, all-purpose flour, cinnamon, baking powder, baking soda and allspice with a whisk until blended. Add to the wet mixture, stirring until smooth. Divide the batter evenly between the prepared pans and bake for 25 minutes or until a toothpick inserted in the center comes out clean. Cool the cakes in the pan slightly, then remove to a rack and cool completely. Remove the parchment paper.

Cream Cheese Frosting:
Beat the cream cheese and butter together until smooth. Gradually add the icing sugar, beating until it reaches a spreadable consistency. Chill for 15 minutes before icing cake.

To assemble the cake:

Set the bottom layer on a plate, pedestal or cake board. Cover with a quarter of the icing and carefully spread half the marmalade over top (if using). Repeat with the second layer. Top with the third cake layer and use the remaining icing to completely cover the cake, swirling decoratively as desired.

Winter Rhubarb Shortcake

Recipe Makeover: Unlike traditional shortcake recipes that use a cake-like biscuit, these sweet oat biscuits have a soluble fiber boost and are low in fat.

Makes 8 shortcakes

A sweet vanilla-speckled biscuit topped with custard and tangy rhubarb. Save the extra rhubarb sauce to serve over ice cream or frozen yogurt.

Stewed Rhubarb:

5 cups	fresh (or frozen unsweetened) chopped rhubarb	1.25 L
1 cup	lightly packed brown sugar	250 mL
2 tbsp	fresh orange juice (approx.)	30 mL

Vanilla Oat Biscuits:

1³/₄ cups	all-purpose flour	425 mL
³/₄ cup	whole-wheat flour	175 mL
¹/₂ cup	old-fashioned rolled oats	125 mL
2 tbsp	granulated sugar	30 mL
1 tbsp	baking powder	15 mL
¹/₂ tsp	salt	2 mL
1 tbsp	finely grated orange peel	15 mL
¹/₃ cup	cold butter, cubed	75 mL
1	vanilla bean or 2 tsp (10 mL) vanilla	1
1 cup	warm milk	250 mL

Custard:

2 cups	skim milk	500 mL
3 tbsp	custard powder	45 mL
3 tbsp	granulated sugar	45 mL

Stewed Rhubarb:

Combine rhubarb, brown sugar and orange juice in a large saucepan. Bring to the boil and simmer until thickened, adding more orange juice if necessary.

Vanilla Oat Biscuits:

Preheat oven to 425°F (220°C). Combine the all-purpose flour, whole-wheat flour, oats, sugar, baking powder, salt and orange peel in a large bowl. Cut in cold butter, using a pastry blender or two knives, until mixture resembles coarse oatmeal. Cut vanilla bean in half and scrape the seeds into the milk. Stir the milk into the flour mixture until a ragged dough forms.

Turn onto a lightly floured surface and knead gently, just until dough comes together. Roll or pat into a round ³/₄-inches (2 cm) thick. Cut with a 3-inch (7.5 cm) round cutter into 8 rounds and place on an ungreased cookie sheet. Any additional dough can be formed into biscuits by hand and saved for another purpose. Bake the biscuits in the preheated oven for 12 to 15 minutes or until golden. Cool.

Custard:
Combine the milk, custard powder and sugar in a microwave-safe bowl.
Microwave on high for 3 to 4 minutes or until thickened, stirring
occasionally. (Or bring the mixture to the boil in a heavy saucepan set over
medium heat, stirring often. Simmer, stirring constantly, until thickened.)

To assemble the shortcakes:
Carefully cut each biscuit in half. Place the bottom halves on the serving
plates. Top each with about ¼ cup (60 mL) of the warm custard and a
spoonful of the rhubarb sauce. Top with the second half of the biscuit and
drizzle a little more rhubarb sauce on top.

TIP: To cut back on the sugar content of the sauce, substitute frozen
strawberries for half the rhubarb and use ½ cup (125 mL) brown sugar
instead of 1 cup (250 mL).

Raspberry, Mango and Kiwi Cheesecake

PER SERVING	
Calories	389
Fat (g)	22
Protein (g)	7
Carbohydrate (g)	43
Fiber (g)	4
Sodium (mg)	187

A high source of fiber. An excellent source of vitamin A and vitamin D.

Recipe Makeover: This beautiful showpiece cheesecake gets its fiber boost from the whole-wheat shortbread crust and the gorgeous glazed fruit topping.

Serves 12

Delicious and creamy with a beautiful glazed fruit top. Fresh raspberries are essential for this recipe, so try it during berry season.

Crust:

1 cup	whole-wheat flour	250 mL
1/4 cup	ground almonds	60 mL
1/2 cup	lightly packed brown sugar	125 mL
1/3 cup	cold butter, cubed	75 mL

Filling:

16 oz	light brick-style cream cheese, softened	500 g
2/3 cup	granulated sugar	150 mL
2	eggs	2
1 tsp	finely grated lime peel	5 mL
1 tbsp	fresh lime juice	15 mL
1/2 cup	sour cream	125 mL

Topping:

1	mango, peeled and chopped	1
1 tbsp	granulated sugar	15 mL
2 tsp	fresh lime juice	10 mL
3	kiwis, peeled and sliced	3
1 1/2 cups	fresh raspberries	375 mL
1/4 cup	seedless raspberry jam, melted	60 mL

Crust:

Preheat the oven to 325°F (160°C). Stir the flour with the almonds and brown sugar. Using a pastry blender or fork, cut in the cold butter until the mixture resembles coarse oatmeal. Press the crumbs into the bottom of a 9-inch (2.5 L) springform pan. Bake in the preheated oven for 15 minutes or until lightly golden. Cool to room temperature.

Filling:

Beat the cream cheese with an electric mixer until very smooth. Add the sugar and beat until well combined. Add the eggs one at a time, scraping down the sides of the bowl between additions. Add the lime peel, juice and sour cream and blend on low, just until combined. Pour on top of the crust. Bake at 325°F (160°C) for 40 minutes or until just set. Run a thin knife around the edge of the cheesecake. Cool to room temperature, then cool completely in the refrigerator (at least 6 hours or overnight).

Topping:

Process the mango with the sugar and lime juice in a food processor until smooth. Spread the mango mixture over the surface of the cheesecake. Place the kiwi slices in a ring around the edge of the top of the cheesecake. Arrange the raspberries inside the ring to cover the surface. Carefully brush the fruit with the melted jam and chill for 30 minutes to set.

To serve, remove the outer ring of the pan and slice the cheesecake with a sharp knife. Have a wet paper towel handy to clean the knife between slices for the best presentation.

Bread Pudding Semi-Freddo

Serves 10

PER SERVING

Calories	354
Fat (g)	22
Protein (g)	7
Carbohydrate (g)	37
Fiber (g)	3
Sodium (mg)	166

A source of fiber. An excellent source of vitamin D.

Try this decadent dessert just once, and it will become a family favorite. Inspired by homey bread pudding, it has an elegant touch when frozen. Keeping a fancy dessert like this in the freezer is the perfect way to eliminate rush during the entertaining season.

2 cups	coarse fresh whole-wheat breadcrumbs (about 3 slices of bread)	500 mL
2 tbsp	melted butter	30 mL
2 tbsp	brown sugar	30 mL
3	egg yolks	3
$^2/_3$ cup	granulated sugar	150 mL
1 tbsp	dark rum or 1 tsp (5 mL) vanilla	15 mL
1 tbsp	ground cinnamon	15 mL
$^1/_4$ tsp	salt	1 mL
1 cup	whipping (35%) cream	250 mL
1 cup	smooth ricotta cheese, light if preferred	250 mL
1 cup	toasted chopped pecans	250 mL
1 cup	sultana raisins	250 mL

Preheat the oven to 325°F (160°C). Toss the breadcrumbs with the butter and brown sugar and spread on a foil-lined baking sheet. Bake the crumbs for 15 minutes until golden and toasted, stirring once during baking. Cool the crumbs completely, then crumble finely.

In a large heatproof bowl set over simmering water, whisk the egg yolks with the sugar, rum, cinnamon and salt until thick and heated through, about 2 minutes. Remove the bowl from the heat and cover with a piece of plastic wrap that covers the surface. Chill until cool.

In a chilled bowl, beat the whipping cream with an electric mixer until very thick. Gently fold into the chilled egg mixture along with the ricotta cheese, pecans and raisins.

Line a 9- × 5-inch (2 L) loaf pan with plastic wrap, allowing extra to hang over the edge. Sprinkle in a quarter of the crumb mixture. Spoon in a third of the cream mixture, smoothing the top. Repeat the layers twice and sprinkle with the remaining crumbs. Freeze until firm, at least 6 hours or up to 1 week. Thaw at room temperature for 10 minutes before slicing with a serrated knife.

TIP: To make breadcrumbs, pulse bread in a blender or food processor until crumbly.

Maple, Pear and Walnut Slice

Serves 10

Similar to apple crisp, this dessert is lovely served with a scoop of vanilla ice cream or frozen yogurt.

PER SERVING	
Calories	473
Fat (g)	19
Protein (g)	7
Carbohydrate (g)	75
Fiber (g)	7
Sodium (mg)	175

A very high source of fiber. An excellent source of vitamin D and magnesium.

Crust:

1/2 cup	softened butter	125 mL
1 cup	granulated sugar	250 mL
2 cups	whole-wheat flour	500 mL
1 tbsp	ground cinnamon	15 mL
pinch	salt	pinch

Filling:

6	pears, peeled and chopped	6
1 tbsp	fresh lemon juice	15 mL
1/2 cup	maple syrup	125 mL

Topping:

1/4 cup	brown sugar	60 mL
1/2 cup	rolled oats, large flake	125 mL
1/2 cup	chopped walnuts, toasted	125 mL
1/4 cup	melted butter	60 mL

Crust:
Preheat the oven to 350°F (180°C). Blend the butter with the sugar until creamy. Blend in the flour, cinnamon and salt until crumbly and press into a 9- × 13-inch (3 L) glass baking dish. Bake on the lower rack in the oven for 10 minutes or until pale gold.

Filling:
Toss the pears with the lemon juice and maple syrup. Spread over the pastry base.

Topping:
Blend the brown sugar with the oats and walnuts, stir in the butter and sprinkle evenly over the pears. Bake for 45 minutes or until pears are tender. Broil on high for 2 to 3 minutes or until the topping is golden.

Sensational Sauces: Fiber-Boosted Ice Cream Toppings

A sundae does not need to be a wasted extravagance. Top your ice cream or low-fat frozen yogurt with one of these delicious sauces that provide more fiber than typical chocolate and caramel sauces.

PER SERVING (¼ cup)	
Calories	78
Fat (g)	0
Protein (g)	0
Carbohydrate (g)	20
Fiber (g)	2
Sodium (mg)	1
A source of fiber.	

Wild Blueberry-Orange Sauce
Makes 1½ cups (375 mL)

A rich and luscious sauce that comes conveniently out of your freezer.

2 cups	frozen wild blueberries	500 mL
½ cup	granulated sugar	125 mL
2 tsp	cornstarch	10 mL
¼ cup	fresh orange juice	60 mL
1 tbsp	finely grated orange peel	15 mL
1 tbsp	orange liqueur such as Grand Marnier (optional)	15 mL

Combine the blueberries, sugar, cornstarch and orange juice in a saucepan set over medium heat. Bring to a boil and reduce the heat. Simmer until slightly thickened. Stir in the orange peel and liqueur, if using. Serve warm or store in the refrigerator until ready to use (up to 5 days).

PER SERVING (¼ cup)	
Calories	274
Fat (g)	12
Protein (g)	1
Carbohydrate (g)	45
Fiber (g)	2
Sodium (mg)	130
A source of fiber. An excellent source of vitamin D.	

Spicy Mango-Lime Caramel Sauce
Makes about 1½ cups (375 mL)

Although unconventional, the hot pepper sauce adds a unique and delicious dimension to this exotic topping.

¼ cup	butter	60 mL
2	mangos, peeled and finely chopped (to make about 2 cups)	2
½ cup	lightly packed brown sugar	125 mL
1 tsp	finely grated lime peel	5 mL
1 tbsp	fresh lime juice	15 mL
1 tsp	hot pepper sauce (optional)	5 mL

Melt the butter in a saucepan set over medium heat. Add the mangos and cook until lightly browned, about 3 minutes. Add brown sugar, stirring until dissolved, and cook for 2 minutes, until the sauce thickens slightly. Remove from heat and stir in the lime peel, juice and hot pepper sauce if using. Serve warm or reserve in refrigerator up to 3 days until ready to use. Reheat in microwave or in a saucepan before serving.

Winter Fruit Sauce
Makes 2 cups (500 mL)

An elegant dried-fruit compote that can also be served at breakfast with yogurt and oatmeal or granola.

2 cups	mixed coarsely chopped dried fruit such as apples, pears, apricots and peaches	500 mL
1/4 cup	dried sour cherries	60 mL
1 tbsp	dried blueberries	15 mL
1 1/4 cups	white grape or cranberry juice	300 mL
1/2 cup	granulated sugar	125 mL
1	cinnamon stick	1

Combine the mixed dried fruit, cherries, blueberries and juice in a non-reactive bowl or pot. Let the fruit stand, covered, at room temperature for 4 hours or overnight to plump it up. Stir in the sugar and cinnamon stick and bring the mixture to the boil. Reduce the heat and simmer for 10 minutes or until the fruit is tender and the liquid thickened. Serve warm or hold in the refrigerator for up to 1 week or in the freezer for up to 2 months.

Variation:
For a different flavor, replace the cinnamon stick with one vanilla bean cut in half lengthwise. After simmering the fruit, remove the vanilla bean and scrape the seeds into the fruit. Stir to combine.

PER SERVING (1/4 cup)	
Calories	143
Fat (g)	0
Protein (g)	1
Carbohydrate (g)	37
Fiber (g)	3
Sodium (mg)	7
A source of fiber.	

Three-Week Fiber-Boosting Plan

It is important to add fiber to your diet gradually to make it easier for your digestive system to handle the influx of fruit, vegetables, whole grains and legumes. Following a three-week plan will allow your body to become accustomed to fiber-rich foods and minimize unpleasant side effects such as bloating and gas.

This checklist involves taking a look at your typical eating habits so you become aware of the shortfalls in your current diet. Changes that start in the supermarket and carry on through to the table will help you develop healthy eating habits. By the end of the three weeks, you should have a new routine of eating nutritious high-fiber foods with every meal.

Week 1

Before making any changes to your routine, compile a three-day record of everything you eat. Write down what you eat at breakfast, lunch and dinner. Don't forget to include snacks. Compare your diet to *Canada's Food Guide to Healthy Eating* or *The American Food Guide Pyramid*. The guides show examples of foods and typical serving sizes in each category. Things to watch for include:

1. Are you eating enough servings of fruits and vegetables?
2. Are you eating enough grain products? What grains are you eating more often?
3. Are you eating enough meats and meat alternatives? How often do you include legumes as a meat alternative?
4. Are you including dairy products or other calcium sources in your diet?

✔ Do a pantry audit: What foods do you keep on hand, and where could you make some healthful changes?

✔ Start by making one or two small changes each day, for example:

Day 1: Eat a whole orange instead of drinking a glass of orange juice in the morning.

Day 2: Have your sandwich at lunch on whole-wheat bread instead of white.

Day 3: Add legumes to one of your meals. For example, make chili or have baked beans as a side dish.

Day 4: Snack on fresh vegetables such as carrots and celery sticks or eat an apple instead of reaching for a Danish or a cookie when hunger strikes.

Day 5: Plan your supper around the vegetables instead of the meat. Have a meatless stir-fry or a veggie-rich soup for a change.

✔ Be sure to drink at least 6 to 8 glasses of water a day.

Week 2

On the basis of the pantry audit in Week 1, create a shopping list to stock fiber-rich foods to have on hand for quick meal solutions. Some ideas include:

- Whole-wheat pastas such as spaghetti, rotini and macaroni
- Whole grains such as brown and wild rice, quinoa, couscous and barley for side dishes
- Hearty breads such as whole-wheat, pumpernickel and rye
- Other whole-wheat items such as pitas, tortillas and English muffins
- Canned legumes such as baked beans, kidney beans, chickpeas and lentils
- Dried fruit such as apple rings, dates, figs, dried cranberries, raisins and apricots
- Nuts and seeds such as unblanched almonds, peanuts, pecans, sesame seeds and pumpkin seeds for recipes and snacking
- Hearty root vegetables such as potatoes, sweet potatoes, parsnips and carrots.
- Frozen or canned vegetables such as corn, peas, broccoli, spinach and green beans
- Frozen loose-pack berries such as blueberries, raspberries, strawberries and cranberries

Check out the Fiber Boosters charts on pages 12–14 for more ideas.

✔ Make changes in two meals each day to incorporate higher-fiber foods.

Breakfast time is a good place to start, since there are so many natural choices of whole-grain cereals, breads, bagels and muffins. Start the day with foods that provide lasting energy such as oatmeal, or boost your vitamin intake with a fruit salad.

Lunches are often just thrown together in the morning, so plan ahead and pack a healthy lunch the night before. Marinated salads keep well and can be served with a crusty whole-wheat roll.

At supper, fiber can be found in side dishes such as potatoes with the skins on, whole-wheat pasta and salads.

✔ Drink a minimum of 6 to 8 glasses of water a day, drinking more as you add more fiber to your meals.

Week 3

With your family's help, if possible, plan your menu for the week. Have fun looking through this book and choosing recipes to try. When planning breakfasts and lunches, consider foods that are quick and easy to prepare or that pack well.

Check out the following five-day meal plan for ideas (recipes in *Fiber Boost* are in italics):

Day	Breakfast	Lunch	Dinner
1	*Mix-and-Match Oatmeal Bowls* Fruit Juice with Pulp	*Hummus Salad All-in-One Muffin*	Roast chicken or broiled chicken breasts *Smashed Potatoes Chili-Lime Corn Skillet*
2	*Daily Detox Smoothies*	Chicken-salad sandwich in a whole-wheat pita	*Heart-Healthy Minestrone* Crusty whole-wheat rolls
3	Toasted bagel with *Orange-Chocolate Fig Spread*	*Heart-Healthy Minestrone* Crusty wheat rolls	*Harvest Pork and Root-Vegetable Supper*
4	Whole orange or grapefruit Whole-grain cereal	*Garden Veggie Wrap* Applesauce	*Maple-Stout Meatballs* Brown rice Broccoli spears
5	*All-in-One Muffin* Fruit Salad	Vegetable sticks and Whole-wheat pita wedges with *Hummus*	*Dilly Salmon Pasta Primavera* Tossed salad

✔ Again, remember to drink an adequate amount of non-caffeinated beverages throughout the day so your body will have the fluid it needs to let the fiber work.

Additional Tips:

✔ Make batches of muffins and cookies on weekends or when you have some free time. Individually wrap and freeze to put in lunches or to grab as a snack or dessert.

✔ Use leftovers in your lunch the next day: Leftover chicken becomes chicken salad. Or pack extra soup into containers ready for the lunchbox.

✔ Think of color and variety when planning your meals.

Menu-Planning Guide

Speedy Weeknight Choices (finished in less than 30 minutes)

- Southwestern Supper Salad
- Ginger Chicken Soup with Soba Noodles
- Won't Miss the Meat-Less Chili
- Italian Flag Pasta
- Dilly Salmon Pasta Primavera
- Shrimp and Soba Noodles

Winter Warm-ups: Comforting Family Recipes for Cold Nights

- Heart-Healthy Minestrone
- Won't Miss the Meat-Less Chili
- Undercover Wonder Baked Pasta
- Takin' It Easy Brisket Braise
- Harvest Pork and Root-Vegetable Supper
- Reuben Strata
- Creamy Chicken Cobbler
- Moroccan Chicken and Lentil Stew

Perfect for Potluck

- Maple-Stout Meatballs
- Mango Tango Slaw
- Diva Pasta Salad
- Indian Princess Salad
- Rutabaga, Parsnip and Apple Crumble
- Roasted Fennel and Three Peppers
- Undercover Wonder Baked Pasta
- Reuben Strata
- Pumpernickel Muffaletta

- Bombay Tuna-Stuffed Potatoes
- Gemstone Soda Bread
- Caramel-Apple Sticky Buns
- Mahogany Spice Loaf
- Palm Grove Loaf
- Kitchen Sink Cookies
- Pineapple-Cherry Upside-Down Cake
- Carrot Pineapple Tower Cake
- Raspberry, Mango and Kiwi Cheesecake
- Maple, Pear and Walnut Slice

Special-Occasion Menus

- **Fall Feast: An Elegant Dinner For Eight**
  Roasted Parsnip and Pear Soup
  Orchard Chèvre-Stuffed Pork Loin
  Smashed Potatoes (Roasted Garlic and Apple) double recipe
  Roasted Fennel and Three Peppers
  Winter Rhubarb Shortcake
- **Easy Holiday Supper**
  Cran-Orange-Stuffed Turkey Breast
  Smashed Potatoes Sea Salt and Pepper (double recipe)
  Steamed Carrots
  Sugar-Bush Brussels Sprouts
  Mixed Berry Crunch Trifle
- **Rustic Entertaining for Six**
  Wilted Spinach Salad with Grapefruit and Avocado
  Trattoria Lamb Shanks with Bean Ragout
  Savory Garlic and Herb Spelt Biscuits
  Bread Pudding Semi-Freddo

Contact Information for Health Organizations

Before making any significant dietary change, you should see a health professional such as your family doctor or a public-health dietitian. This book is just a tool to help you cook healthful fiber-rich foods and should not be considered a medical diet. For more information on healthy eating, the following websites and organizations have information available to the public.

Sources of nutrition information in Canada:

Dietitians of Canada
480 University Avenue, Suite 604
Toronto ON M5G 1V2
Tel: 416-596-0857 Fax: 416-596-0603
www.dietitian.ca

Canadian Diabetes Association
National Life Building
1400-522 University Ave
Toronto ON M5G 2R5
1-800-226-8464
www.diabetes.ca

Health Canada
A.L. 0900C2
Ottawa, ON K1A 0K9
Tel: 613-957-2991
**www.hc-sc.gc.ca/hpfb-dgpsa/
onpp-bppn/index.html**

Canadian Cancer Society
National Office
Suite 200, 10 Alcorn Avenue
Toronto ON M4V 3B1
Tel: 416-961-7223
www.cancer.ca

Heart and Stroke Foundation Canada
222 Queen Street, Suite 1402
Ottawa, ON K1P 5V9
Tel: 613-569-4361
Fax: 613-569-3278
www.heartandstroke.ca

Other websites to check out:

National Cancer Institute, U.S.
www.nci.nih.gov

Food and Nutrition Information Center
www.nalusda.gov/fnic

The American Heart Association
www.americanheart.org

American Dietetic Association:
www.eatright.org

American Diabetes Association
www.diabetes.org

World Health Organization
www.who.int/en

Acknowledgments

Greatest thanks to Dana McCauley who inspired me to write *Fiber Boost* and whose kind words start this book. You truly have a generous spirit; not just content with your own success, you take time out of your busy life to pull up those around you. Thank you for being a mentor and good friend.

I am grateful to Anna Porter who first heard my proposal and took a chance on a new author. I would also like to thank Clare McKeon who was involved in the concept and first draft. I sincerely appreciate the whole team at Key Porter, especially my editor Michael Mouland and art director Peter Maher. Praise and thanks goes to Pete Patterson and Julie Zambonelli who made the food look so great. Personal thanks to George Skerratt who took my back cover photo.

Many, many thanks to the team of talented chefs, home economists and cooks who tested the recipes, including Tracey Syvret, Charmaine Broughton, Marian Sweetnam, Adell Shneer, Doug Smith and Joan Snider. I appreciate all of your contributions to the quality of the recipes. Thanks again to Dana for providing a test kitchen and an experienced palate.

More thanks to my support network, starting with my family who has always been there for me with love and encouragement. (My most devoted taster has always been my dad!) I also appreciate all of the kind words and enthusiasm from my "girls", my extended family at St. Andrew's and many friends in my hometown of Lindsay. Further thanks to my professors at Brescia College at U.W.O. for a great nutritional grounding with a special mention to Dr. Elizabeth Bright-See and Dr. Leonard Piché for additional advice during the writing of *Fiber Boost*.

It has been a wonderful experience watching *Fiber Boost* come together. I hope that everyone will enjoy cooking from it as much as I enjoyed writing it.

Index